Green Smoothie
CLEANSE

Green Smoothie
CLEANSE

Detox, Lose Weight and Restore Your Health
with the World's Most Powerful Superfoods

Lisa Sussman

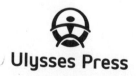

Ulysses Press

Published in the U.S. by:
Ulysses Press
P.O. Box 3440
Berkeley, CA 94703
www.ulyssespress.com

ISBN13: 978-1-61243-267-0
Library of Congress Control Number: 2013947586

Printed in Canada by Marquis Book Printing

Acquisitions Editor: Keith Riegert
Managing Editor: Claire Chun
Editor: Lauren Harrison
Proofreader: Elyce Berrigan-Dunlop
Index: Sayre Van Young
Cover Design: what!design @ whatweb.com
Cover art: © vanillaechoes/shutterstock.com
Design and Layout: Jake Flaherty
Interior art from shutterstock.com: pages 6, 40, 105, 111, 180, 189 © Morphart Creation; pages 13, 54, 94, 122, 141, 201 © Hein Nouwens; page 25 © Shlapak Liliya; page 62 © Arafel; page 160 © rudall30; page 169 © Margarita Tkachenko

10 9 8 7 6 5 4 3 2 1

Distributed by Publishers Group West

Contents

PART I

CLEANSING
MATTERS

• •

"Let food be thy medicine and medicine be thy food."

—Hippocrates

CHAPTER ONE

Why Cleanse with Smoothies?

First things first: Let's all get on the same page about what we're calling a cleanse. This is important because not all cleanse and/or detox programs are created equal. There are those that last a day, others that are a few days or weeks, and some that are months long. Some target specific illnesses while others are limited to organic foods, and then there are a few that include no food at all (and, frankly, aren't all that different from the type of fast you might be forced to adopt if you were stranded on a desert island).

The green smoothie cleanse does not fall into any of those categories, per se. For instance, if you have a chronic illness, it may make you feel better and healthier, but no one is claiming that chugging spinach and carrots for a week will cure you. Also, rather than adhering to a strict, limited timeline, how long you cleanse is completely up to you, your schedule, and your lifestyle. There's a green smoothie cleanse to fit your every need. And none of these are "let's starve ourselves and live on spicy lemonade for a month" plans, so you'll never suffer from hungry pangs during that time, even if you follow the two-week cleanse. While you may certainly feel lightheaded, dizzy, or nauseous, it quickly passes and you won't experience intense levels that you would on a no-food "cleanse." Nor will you feel as if you were recovering from the mother of all hangovers.

One of These Things Isn't Like the Other

There's a bountiful difference between cleansing and detoxing. Here's the skinny on both, and even this is open to interpretation, depending on whom you're talking to. But generally:

A CLEANSE...	A DETOX ...
Will clear and clean up the digestive tract (think from mouth to anus) of toxins, compacted fecal matter, bacteria, and fungi	Will eliminate environmental toxins that the body absorbs or ingests in day-to-day living, such as cigarette smoke, pollution, chemicals found in cleaning products, and so on
Ups your daily dose of veggies and fruits to boost fiber and help with the clean-out	Decreases or even eliminates your intake of all foods
Is a holistic, long-term approach to put the body in balance by feeding it the fuel it needs to function at its best	Is a quick fix to target a specific imbalance

Frankly, we rarely need the kind of complete industrial vacuum clear-out of a detox diet. Yes, our world is filled with environmental pollutants and toxins with names so long and unpronounceable that they look like a text gone haywire when written down. But a healthy liver and kidneys will do a fine job of detoxifying the body on a daily basis.

For all you OCD-types, a green smoothie cleanse won't extract that piece of gum you swallowed in first grade that's still stuck to your intestinal lining. (But only because it's now a gum tree growing in your stomach. OK, truth is your body ejected that wad long ago. Gum is of little value to the body and because of its makeup it passes through slower than most foodstuffs, but eventually the normal housekeeping waves in the digestive tract will sort of push it through, and it will come out pretty unmolested).

For all those instant-gratification types, know that going on a green smoothie cleanse won't make you lose 20 pounds in one day. (Anyway, chances are the only thing you're shedding when you do one of those total deprivation detoxes is water weight, which will pour back on once you start eating again.)

For all the "ewww get these toxins out of my body types," the green smoothie cleanse will not leave your digestive tract Windex clean—nor should it. The fact is, the kind of irrigation that hoses your colon can end up throwing the baby out with the bathwater. Scientists used to think that the only good microbe was a dead one. But our bodies are full of bacteria, fungi, viruses, and other microbes that we can't live without, to the point that doctors are performing fecal transplants for some people with life-threatening infections with the bacterium *Clostridium difficile* to replace their ailing microbes with a colony of healthy ones.

The plus side, however, is what you'll feel after going on a green smoothie cleanse: re-energized, recharged, and revitalized. Rather than a complete clear-out, the green smoothie cleanse is more about resetting your metabolism, digestion, and palate. With each drink, you're rebooting your body to get on a healthy-eating and -living track.

What we do need is lots of good old-fashioned fiber to help these organs rid our bodies of whatever waste we accumulate. Because truth be told, the biggest threat to preventing our bodies from functioning at optimum is the processed crap that we freely put in our mouths, chew up, and swallow. Call it SAD, aka the Standard American Diet of fast (read "fat") and convenience foods. Science today has proven over and over again that eating a healthy diet full of vegetables and fruit nourishes our bodies and keeps our immune systems fighting strong against illness, infection, and disease.

Bite Me!

In an ideal world, eating rather than drinking an apple or a bowl of naked greens is the better option.

A plateful of kale and strawberries may make more of a mental impact than a mashed-up glass of these ingredients. But it's always going to be easier to glug down 500 calories of fruits and vegetables than chew them.

Studies show that chewing food makes you feel fuller faster than drinking that exact same food in blended form. This means that you end up ingesting fewer calories when you chew your food. It seems it takes about 20 minutes for the "I'm full! Stop eating right this minute!" signals sent from your gut reach your brain. Which is fine, as a sit-down, cut-and-chew meal generally lasts at least that long. But it only takes a few minutes to down a smoothie, so you're inevitably going to be done waaay before your brain receives its stop and desist satiation message.

However, few of us are lucky to live in that ideal of a slow-lane world where we regularly have the time to leisurely linger at the table over a Martha Stewart–worthy platter of fruits and veggies. The average person's day is so busy that few have the time to even peel a cucumber, let alone take 20 minutes to nibble it.

And that is the appeal of drinking. It isn't impossible to drink nine servings of fruits and vegetables (aka 4.5 cups) a day—or even in a few hours.

This isn't to say that smoothies should completely replace eating solid foods. That isn't what they are meant to do. But they can be a supplement to your daily diet by helping you eat more vegetables and fruit and, when needed, are a healthy way to cleanse and jumpstart a healthier lifestyle.

Smooth Move

To juice or to blend isn't the question when it comes to cleansing. The short and sweet of it is that there's loads of fiber in a green smoothie and there's zero fiber in juices. Which means that there's no way are you going to get those recommended 25 grams (for women) to 38 grams (for men) of the stuff if you opt to liquefy your fruits and veg. If rodents like rabbits or hamsters don't chew on enough high-fiber foods daily, their teeth—which constantly regenerate—may grow uncontrollably and pierce the roof of their mouth, knifing the base their brain. While your choppers—and your brain—are safe, there's no getting around the fact that fiber is the backbone of a good cleanse. Think of it as a nutritional scouring pad:

- Fiber binds with the toxins. This is going to help to push those undesirables out of your body as waste.
- Fiber makes bathroom time easier. When you don't have enough fiber, you don't hit the porcelain basin as often as you probably should and you're therefore at a much higher risk of constipation or, at the very least, some very uncomfortable bowel movements.
- Fiber helps you keep your seat. A high-fiber diet may help to lower your risk of developing hemorrhoids and small pouches in your colon (which can be a sign of diverticular disease and result in crampy pain or discomfort in the lower abdomen, bloating, and constipation).
- Fiber might just keep you alive longer. Pass over the fiber and research shows that you may be opening yourself up to a slew of different cancers, including colon and colorectal. You also raise your risk of heart disease by as much as 40 percent.
- Fiber can prevent a sugar high. Fiber can slow the absorption of sugar and help improve blood sugar levels. This is especially good news for people who have diabetes, as is the research that shows that a healthy diet that includes insoluble fiber may also reduce the risk of developing type 2 diabetes.
- Fiber can help you fit into your favorite pants. High-fiber foods generally require more chewing time, which gives your body time to register when you're no longer hungry, so you're less likely to overeat. In smoothies, a high-fiber diet tends to make a "meal" feel larger, so you end up staying fuller for a greater amount of time. And high-fi-

ber diets also tend to be less "energy dense," which means they have fewer calories for the same volume of food. Some fibers may also stimulate CCK, an appetite-suppressing hormone in the gut.

- Fiber can improve your lifestyle. In what may be for some a fate-worse-than-death, the odds of becoming not only fat but also impotent are increased when fiber isn't on the menu daily. (The fate of the rodent doesn't seem like the worst possible one now, does it?)

This makes total sense. Eat more plants, especially leafy greens. Everyone tells us that—doctors, nutritionists and healthy food gurus like Michael Pollan and Mark Bittman, as well as hale and hearty celebrity eaters such as Gwyneth Paltrow, Drew Barrymore, Olivia Wilde, Gisele Bündchen, Miranda Kerr, Nicole Richie, Fergie, Amanda Seyfried, Eva Longoria, Hillary Duff, and Vanessa Hudgens, Channing Tatum, Owen Wilson, Josh Duhamel, and Ryan Seacrest, to name-drop just a few. In fact, some doctors are now even putting their money—well, their scrip pads—where their mouth is. In a program initiated in New York, physicians are prescribing vegetables and fruit to at-risk families where obesity is causing a health concern.

Green is the new black in the food world. The only problem is that leafy, vitamin-pumped veggies and fruits just don't tend to be the kind of foods we crave. We especially don't crave the nine servings—which measures out at around 4½ cups—of fruits and vegetables that the Harvard School of Public Health recommends we eat daily. In fact, most of us don't even come close. No wonder, as it's hard to find enough room on your plate for that much plant life.

The solution? Simple: Put them in your glass!

By making the switch from the typical SAD eating to drinking high-fiber and nutrient-dense foods, you'll give your body the opportunity to "rest and digest." This sounds like a modest goal, but it really is the key to good health.

Green smoothies are as close to a perfect meal as you can get—delicious, nutritious, and fast. Since they are blended into a liquid form that breaks down the plant, your body absorbs the benefits of the fiber more efficiently than it would with chewing. Blending also makes it easier for your body to digest the fiber and nutrients. One last thing: Your liquid salad comes without the dressings, croutons, and bacon bits that turn a basic, garden-variety salad into a chlorophyll donut. Win, win, win.

Bon appétit! Or, to be more accurate, should that be "Bottoms up"?!

CHAPTER TWO

What *Is* That Sludge?

Before we start, let's just clarify one thing: Today's green smoothie isn't your groovy, tie-dyed hippie smoothie left over from the 1960s. The first commercial smoothies, marketed as a healthy dairy alternative to sugary sodas, were made with milk, yogurt, or ice cream with some fruits and maybe even chocolate or peanut butter with a dollop of wheat germ, brewer's yeast, or whey to give them the illusion of being healthy.

Though they certainly were a better alternative to chugging a soda (which was at the same time rapidly establishing itself as the beverage America would like to teach the world to drink), these early smoothies were still chock-full of fat and sugar and don't even begin to compare to the benefits of today's lean, clean green smoothies.

Still, no one—except for the true green smoothie convert, aka The Greenster (you can recognize them by their permanent green mustaches)—is claiming for a minute that a green smoothie is a pretty thing. A glassful of verdant (or, more likely if you're a newbie blender, grayish-brownish olive) liquid isn't exactly the Iron Chef kind of presentation that's going to make a person smack their lips and say, "I want to get me some of that." If anything, your typical green smoothie will probably initially conjure memories of Mom force-feeding you mushy broccoli and peas. Yum.

Sure, there are those delightful vibrant-green packaged concoctions available everywhere from your local health food store to the global big-box supermarket. But like many commercialized foods, the store-bought smoothie is like its earlier incarnation in that it's often weighed down by more fat, sugar, and calories than its healthy appearance might suggest. Some have little or no fiber at all. The first ingredient is often a fruit juice like apple, or even fruit sorbet to sweeten the look and taste. While there's nothing wrong with fruit as one of your smoothie ingredients, apple juice does not have enough nourishment to even keep the doctor away. The primary liquid should be plain, old-fashioned water—or, if you want to get fancy, coconut water. In addition, there needs to be a healthy dose of greens in order to make sure you're getting the full hale and hearty impact with each sip.

That said, green smoothies can and do taste a lot better than they look and, with practice and the right recipe, can even be blended to look as good as they taste. That is where the fruit struts its stuff. Their natural sweetness stops your green smoothie from tasting "too" green.

All you need to do is memorize a simple ratio of 60 percent fruit to 40 percent greens. In other words, for every 3 cups of fruit, add 1 cup of greens. Sure, hardcore Greensters will advocate a reverse of that ratio—60 percent greens to 40 percent fruit—but even Popeye might have a hard time gulping that much raw green stuff. As you get more adept at blending and figuring out which combos tickle your taste buds, you might get bolder and up that to an even 50:50 ratio.

Still, it's hard to believe that this thing isn't only not going to taste like liquid grass, but that it's actually going to taste *good*. Upfront and truthfully, there's no disputing that some of the vegetables in their raw state tend to taste bitter and downright unpleasant. Kale, anyone? But a green smoothie isn't like a shot of wheatgrass juice (which, sadly, never tastes like anything but a glass of wheatgrass juice). Something magical happens when the bitter greens are atomized into a pulpy liquid. Like a cocoa bean once it becomes a Hershey's Kiss, kale, when chopped up with other vegetables and greens, suddenly has an almost sweet aftertaste that makes it a mighty tasty way to pack in a lot of nutrients like iron and vitamin K (which, sadly, cannot be found in any of your favorite foods like airline peanuts, wine, fried Oreos, or movie popcorn). Also, once you find some recipes that work for you, you'll probably barely taste if the veggies have a slightly bitter side because the sweet flavor of the fruit tends to dominate the drink's flavor, while the greens balance out the fruit's sweetness, adding a tasty, zesty punch.

The main thing is to not overthink it and get too tied to your ratio because the fruit/vegetable balance you end up with is going to ultimately depend on the kind of greens you're using at the moment. Some, like kale and mustard, have a strong, spicy flavor while others, like collards or spinach, have a milder taste. The only real hard and fast rule is that you can throw in less or no fruit at all, but never add more than 60 percent. This keeps your green smoothie from spilling out of the health-shake category and into the sweet-snack-shake one.

Another thing to remember is that while all greens are veggies, not all veggies are greens. The USDA organizes vegetables into five subgroups based on their nutrient content. Read carefully, as the list would challenge even a nutritionist:

1. **Dark Green:** These are mostly leafy, such as collards, kale, dark green leafy lettuces such as romaine and mesclun greens, bok choy, and spinach, but this category also includes broccoli just to keep you on your toes.

2. **Starchy:** As expected, this is where you'll find corn, green peas, potatoes, and cassava, but also, surprisingly, items commonly thought of as fruits, such as plantains and green bananas, are also categorized here.

3. **Red & Orange** (the amerpsand is the USDA's attempt at vegetable whimsy): Carrots & sweet potatoes & the confusing are-

they-fruits-or-vegetables acorn & butternut squashes, pumpkin, red peppers, & tomatoes (see Chew on This, page 52).

4. **Beans and Peas:** Black beans, chickpeas, lentils, soy beans, navy beans, kidney beans, and split peas—in short, the gassy category.

5. **Others** (aka the stuff your mother could never convince you to eat): Artichokes, asparagus, avocado (although to make it even more confusing, these are actually fruit; see Chew On This, page 52), bean sprouts, beets, Brussels sprouts, cabbage, cauliflower, celery, cucumbers, eggplant, green beans, green peppers, iceberg lettuce, mushrooms, okra, onions, and zucchini covers most of them.

So that is your typical nuclear vegetable family (see the next chapter for info on how to know, in fewer than 20 questions, if something is a fruit, vegetable, or grain).

To qualify for a green smoothie, the vegetables should come out of the first category or, to sound a bit like a Match.com personal ad, be dark, green, and leafy. That isn't to say that the remaining veggies should be thrown on the compost heap. Some (usually the kind that are botanically fruits, such as red peppers and tomatoes; see Chew On This, page 52) make tasty additions—and even sweeter extras than green vegetables like broccoli or Brussels sprouts. But they don't count as part of the 40 percent ratio.

While it's best to keep things simple initially, there are flavor additives that get the Green Smoothie Seal of Approval. Protein powders and protein, nuts, seeds, superfoods like cacao (which is a healthier—and therefore more expensive—way of saying cocoa) and goji berries, herbs and spices, natural sweeteners such as stevia and honey, and even some dairy products like yogurt and kefir are all ingredients that can give your smoothie a flavor boost and sometimes even rank up its nutritional and health gains (see Add-Ins, page 211).

What has probably become obvious by now is that the ratio and ingredient requirements of a truly healthy green smoothie are hard to control when you're buying your smoothies from an outside source; this is why it really is better to make them yourself from scratch. Only then can you know exactly what you're getting in each and every glass. After all, if you're going to make the effort of going on a cleanse, doesn't it make sense to also make the effort to do it right?

The end result, whichever recipe you choose, is a fairly filling drink. So even if you're not going on a Green Smoothie Cleanse, a 16-ounce glass can almost be a meal in itself. "Almost" because unless you add some protein such as nuts or yogurt, it may fill you up but won't keep you full as long as a square meal. This might sound like just the ticket if you're trying to lose weight, but as any dietitian will tell you, consuming too few calories, especially if they come mainly from foods low in protein, actually has a backlash effect on your goal because it causes your body to go into panic mode (i.e., "Where is my next meal coming from?!") and store every available calorie.

The bottom line is that you can do too much of anything—even healthy things. So although you shouldn't live solely on smoothies, you can certainly drink a smoothie or five every day. Greensters will swear that this regular diet of green smoothies gives them more energy, wipes out their junk food cravings, and makes them feel altogether healthier, more optimistic, and kinder toward small animals and children.

While there's no actual scientific basis to these claims, research has confirmed that a regular diet of greens and fruit will help to improve mood, cholesterol levels, and blood pressure and keep diseases such as diabetes, certain cancers, and heart disease at bay... in short, pretty much everything (except maybe cure the economy). Since drinking just one green smoothie a day guarantees that you'll consume your RDA of these foods, then it follows that you reap all the same benefits that you would if you tried to eat that amount of fruits and vegetables—and that you'll also have more time since it's faster to drink than eat nine servings every day. Think liquid gold in a glass.

As to when, the answer is whenever the mood hits you. Some people swear that the morning is the best time to drink a green smoothie because they like starting the day with a verdant boost. Others don't feel comfortable having all that instant fiber on an empty stomach and prefer it as an afternoon pick-me-up, a pre-workout or nighttime snack, or, if they are adding protein, in place of lunch or dinner. Unless you're following a cleanse, which does have a routine, this really is one of those rare whatever-work-best-for-you-that-day things.

Why You Should Drop What You're Doing Right Now and Blend Yourself a Green Smoothie

A green smoothie will make you smarter, stronger, happier, sexier, live longer, and add time to your day. Got your attention?

Good. Here's the disclaimer: You'll be smarter because of how you eat; stronger because you're more likely to follow through on that workout when you eat healthy; happier because whatever the short-term gratification of eating junk food, eating healthy has more long-term effects in the feel-good department; sexier because while an unhealthy diet definitely is a downer on the libido, a healthy one seems to boost it; and younger because eating healthy helps you to live longer and better.

In case that left you hungry for more reasons to drink green, read on:

1. Green smoothies are a no-brainer way to pump up the amount of greens in your diet. Which is easier to eat: a bunch of celery, spinach, kale, and cucumbers or a glass of the same? See? You're smarter already!

2. One word: chlorophyll. Green smoothies are chock-full of the stuff. If you're like most of the world, what you know about

this pigment comes from what you remember from biology class—that chlorophyll is what makes plants green. But some very preliminary research shows that it may help protect healthy people from cancer.

3. Another word: fiber. Green smoothies are also megadoses of fiber. Regular consumption of fiber helps your body's toxic filtration system—i.e., the colon, intestines, kidneys, and liver—work optimally, which helps protect you from certain cancers, diabetes, and weight gain. (Have you ever met a happy constipated person?)

4. A third word: enzymes. Enzymes are specialized proteins that help your body run smoothly, especially its digestion process. Green smoothies contain more live enzymes than any other food.

5. A multisyllabic word: polyphenols. Greens are packed full of them. Research on the effects of dietary polyphenols has found that they can create a firewall against degenerative diseases, particularly cardiovascular diseases and cancers.

6. Two words: free radicals and antioxidants. Free radicals—the bad guys—are the pesky molecules responsible for aging and tissue damage. Green smoothies are bursting with antioxidants—the good guys—which inhibit the deteriorating effect of free radicals, helping to ward off disease and delay aging.

7. A regular diet of green smoothies will make you look mmm-mmm good because they help you snack healthy, which may have a boomerang effect on reducing your processed and junk food cravings, helping you to lose weight and increasing your overall energy. In addition, a nutritionally balanced diet does more than any expensive beauty product for giving you shiny hair, radiant skin, and strong nails.

8. Unlike a diet of salads, consuming greens in the form of a smoothie means lots of good taste with none of the oil, salt, cheese, or other add-ins you might toss in to add a flavor boost to your plate o' greens. So you stay lean without feeling mean because you feel deprived. A quick reality check on those store-bought salads: The Caesar salad with all the fixings at one popular fast food chain actually has more calories than an extra-large size of its fries. In comparison, a typical green smoothie usually averages out at 300 calories (although this can quickly rise if you're piling on the add-ins).

9. Green smoothies are probably the healthiest fast food (as opposed to standard SAD fare) there is. It takes only a few minutes to blend one up and you can pour it in a travel mug and take it anywhere. And unlike a burger and fries, or even a carrot and beet juice, they have a good balance of fiber, vitamins, and protein. Think: an incredibly healthy meal in a cup.

10. Unlike green juices or a balanced meal, both of which can be time-consuming and expensive, a giant smoothie can take less than five minutes to make and clean up and, in the case of juice, uses less produce to get better results.

Disease-Proof Yourself

In case you need any more convincing to get on the green smoothie train, remember that we are what we eat. The body is a sophisticated machine that consistently transforms food for energy and growth. Therefore, eating is being. Over the past 30 years or so, researchers have developed a solid base of science to back up that the way we eat can determine our health. Most of the chronic and degenerative diseases from which we suffer today have a clear-cut link to poor eating habits. Sure, family health history also plays a role in the ultimate manifestation of these illnesses. But diet can trump genes in certain conditions. So while you can't change your genes, you can change what and how you eat, and green smoothies are the perfect way to get back on track.

The Mayo Clinic claims that vegetables and fruit can be the foundation of a person's plan for a healthy life. Not only do vegetables and fruit pack loads of nutrients, but they also fill you up and might prevent you from overeating unhealthy foods. This isn't to say that fruit and vegetables are dietary superheroes, working faster than a speeding bullet, more powerful than a locomotive, and able to conquer all diseases in a single meal. But making certain vegetables and fruit a big part of your daily diet can go a long way to ensuring that you live long and prosper.

TO STOP CARDIOVASCULAR DISEASE COLD

Eat more green leafy vegetables such as lettuce, spinach, Swiss chard, and mustard greens; cruciferous vegetables such as broccoli, cauliflower, cabbage, Brussels sprouts, bok choy, and kale, and citrus fruits such as oranges, lemons, limes, and grapefruits (and their juices).

One glaring fact that came out of the Harvard-based Nurses' Health Study and Health Professionals Follow-up Study, which has followed almost 110,000 men's and women's health and dietary habits for 14 years, is that more is better. Those who munched their way through five servings of vegetables and fruit a day had a 30 percent lower risk of having a heart attack or stroke than those who only managed 1.5 daily servings.

TO STOP HIGH BLOOD PRESSURE COLD

Eat more prunes, watermelon, cantaloupe, avocados, blueberries, raspberries, bananas, apples, pears, apricots, grapefruits, limes, lemons, tangerines, oranges, celery, broccoli, cauliflower, bok choy, cabbage, and Brussels sprouts, spinach, lettuce, kale, mustard greens, Swiss chard, and Chinese cabbage.

High blood pressure is a cause for concern as it can lead to an emergency room full of life-threatening conditions, including heart disease, strokes, kidney failure, and cognitive decline. Blood pressure is also one of the best responders to a healthy diet.

Prunes, avocados, apricots, and especially bananas are packed with potassium, which is essential to maintain blood pressure and cardiac function, and prevent atherosclerosis (clotting of blood in the blood vessels). Lower levels of sodium in the body can help prevent high blood pressure. Avocados are also high in monounsaturated fats, which help to lower LDL or "bad" cholesterol, and increase the level of HDL or "good" cholesterol in the body. These fleshy fruits also contain a fatty alcohol, known as avocadene, which is effective in lowering high blood pressure (though they are also high in calories, so moderation is the key word).

The carotenoids present in melons and the phthalides in celery prevent the hardening and narrowing of the walls of arteries and veins, reducing the chances of constricted flow of blood through the body.

Berries are rich in vitamin C, potassium, fiber, and antioxidants. Blueberries contain a compound known as pterostilbene, which helps in preventing the buildup of plaque in the arteries.

Apples are rich in antioxidants such as vitamin C and flavonoids, which prevent the damage of blood vessels while pears are a good source of antioxidants such as glutathione, which prevents damage of blood vessels. The high pectin content in both of these fruits helps lower cholesterol levels in the body. Citrus fruits are full of vitamin C, phytonutrients, and bioflavonoids, which are anti-inflammatory in nature, and prevent clotting of blood inside the blood vessels. The bioflavonoids, found in the white pith of these fruits, not only help in lowering blood pressure, but also help control cholesterol levels. Cruciferous veggies are high in glutamic acid while leafy greens contain a variety of phytochemicals and antioxidants, like beta-carotene and lutein, which help to fight plaque buildup in the blood vessels, which all helps in lowering blood pressure.

TO STOP CANCERS COLD

Eat more spinach, kale, romaine lettuce, leaf lettuce, mustard greens, collard greens, chicory, broccoli, Swiss chard, pomegranate juice, blueberries, oranges, grapefruit, and tomatoes.

Pomegranate's deep red juice contains polyphenols, isoflavones, and ellagic acid, elements researchers believe make up a potent anti-cancer combo. It has been shown to delay the growth of prostate cancer, stabilize PSA levels in men who have been treated for prostate cancer, and possibly inhibit lung cancer growth.

The pterostilbene found in blueberries has colon cancer–fighting properties. Any fruit rich in vitamin C may reduce the growth of premalignant oral lesions.

Broccoli is a stand-out super cancer-fighting food. It's loaded with vitamin C, beta-carotene, potassium, and a phytochemical called sulphoraphane, which may have anti-prostate and anti-colon cancer properties, as well as the ability to lower the risk of developing bladder cancer.

Green leafy vegetables are excellent sources of fiber, folate, and a wide range of carotenoids such as lutein and zeaxanthin, along with saponins and flavonoids, making them a carcinogen shield to helping reduce chances of developing and/or slow the growth of a variety of cancers: cancer of the mouth, pharynx, and larynx, certain types of breast cancer, ovarian cancer, skin cancer, lung cancer, stomach cancer, colorectal cancer, and prostate cancer.

The lycopene in tomatoes helps neutralize disease-causing free radicals in our bodies, which can prevent prostate cancer and even keep it from becoming more aggressive in those who have already been diagnosed.

TO STOP ASTHMA COLD

Eat more Brussels sprouts.

Brussels sprouts contain high levels of sulforaphane, a compound that increases production of antioxidant enzymes in airways. Those enzymes help prevent inflammation, which leads to diseases like asthma.

TO STOP GASTRIC CONDITIONS COLD

Eat more of pretty much any fruit or vegetable.

One of the superpowers of fruits and vegetables is their indigestible fiber. As fiber passes through the digestive system, it sops up water like a sponge and expands. This can calm the irritable bowel and, by triggering regular bowel movements, can relieve or prevent constipation. That bulking and softening action of insoluble fiber also decreases pressure inside the intestinal tract, which may help prevent diverticulosis (the development of tiny, easily irritated pouches inside the colon) and diverticulitis (the often painful inflammation of these pouches).

TO STOP BAD VISION COLD

Eat more spinach, kale, romaine lettuce, broccoli, carrots, citrus fruits, berries, grapes, red or yellow bell peppers, squash, and kiwi.

Eating certain fruits and vegetables also keeps your eyes in good shape. The vitamin A in carrots and red or yellow bell peppers aids night vision. Dark green leafy vegetables and brightly colored fruit and vegetables contain the substances lutein and zeaxanthin, which protect the retina from damage and may help prevent the development of macular degeneration. Citrus fruits and bell peppers are loaded with vitamin C and flavonoids, which play a role in the prevention of cataracts, macular degeneration, and glaucoma.

CHAPTER THREE

Healthy Eating Rules!

A green and fruity diet is one of the tried-and-true recommendations for the good life. As we've already covered, you will live longer, healthier, and have more energy. The American Institute for Cancer Research has determined that around 40 percent of cancers are diet-related, while studies on diet and nutrition have found that eating lots of greens and fruit can help to actually prevent some of those cancers as well as ward off heart disease and stroke, control blood pressure, avoid a painful intestinal ailment called diverticulitis, and guard against cataract and macular degeneration, two common causes of vision loss.

One thing: What, exactly, does "lots" mean?

The short answer is: a lot more than most of us tend to eat in a day. The Centers for Disease Control and Prevention concluded after an extensive nationwide behavioral study of fruit and vegetable consumption that the average person grazes on a measly total of just three servings or 1½ cups of fruits and vegetables a day (and no, fries don't count in that stat). But dietary guidelines recommend at least five servings or 2½ cups to keep on the robust side of healthy eating, and a minimum of nine or 4½ but preferably 13 servings or 6½ cups of fruits and vegetables a day.

One more thing—although they seem to be as permanently linked as Bert and Ernie, you should actually weigh in with more vegetables than fruit. An in-no-way-set-in-stone ratio is to aim for around 2 cups of vegetables for every cup of fruit. And to make things even more complicated, lettuces and leafy greens actually need to be 1 cup to count as one serving, and ½ cup of dried fruit equals one cup of fruit (see Portion Control, page 27, for more on accepted servings). Finally, what the serving size on the Nutritional Facts label of packaged fruits and vegetables reads isn't necessarily going to be the same size as the ½ cup serving size that the USDA has set for the food pyramid. Some frozen vegetable blends for example may list the serving size as ¾ cup, which would meet one-and-a-half servings of your vegetable need for the day. Call it new math.

Essential Living

While most fruits and vegetables are low in calories and good for your body and overall health, some are definitely a whole lot better than others and offer many more essential nutrients (which is just the official fancy term for describing substances in food that the body needs in order to work properly).

Our bodies need six essential nutrients on a daily basis. These are separated into two groups: macro (carbs, fats, proteins, and water) and micro (vitamins and minerals). (Following the good things come in small packages rule, "micro" doesn't mean that these nutrients aren't important, just that we don't need as much of them as we do of the macros). Last, there's the "other" nutrient (i.e., it isn't officially a nutrient but it's just as essential): fiber or roughage.

The Snap, Crackle, and Pop! of nutrients—protein, carbs, and fat—hog most of the spotlight when it comes to understanding the ingredients of a healthy diet, but fiber is clearly the neglected Pow (those of you who know your breakfast cereal history will recall that Pow, the forgotten fourth Rice Krispies' gnome, was a stand-in for the nutritional value of the popular breakfast cereal).

Portion Control

Life should be easy. And making smoothies should be easier. So here's a quick briefing on what 1 portion (or ½ cup) of fruit or vegetables is roughly equivalent to, according to the USDA:

Fruits

- ½ of a large or 1 small apple, pear, peach, or orange
- ½ of a large or 1 small banana
- 1 smaller fruit such as plums, apricots, kiwis, satsumas, and clementines
- 1 slice or ¼ of a medium cantaloupe
- 1-inch-thick wedge or 6 melon balls of watermelon
- 16 grapes
- 8 large strawberries, raspberries, or cherries
- 2 large tablespoons of fruit salad, stewed fruit, or canned* fruit
- ½ cup of fresh fruit juice
- 1 medium grapefruit
- 1 mango
- 1 large bell pepper
- 1 medium tomato

*Try to find foods "canned" in glass or non-tin containers like Tetra Pak boxes. The resin linings of tin cans have been found to contain bisphenol-A, or BPA, a synthetic estrogen that has been linked to ailments ranging from reproductive problems to heart disease, diabetes, and obesity. Studies show that the BPA in most people's bodies exceeds the amount that suppresses sperm production or causes chromosomal damage to the eggs of animals.

Vegetables

- five 5-inch-long broccoli spears
- ½ of a baked sweet potato
- 1 cup of shredded cabbage
- 2 large stalks of celery
- 10 baby carrots
- 2 medium carrots
- 1 cup of lettuce or raw leafy greens such as spinach, romaine, watercress, endive, and escarole
- ¾ cup (175 ml) of vegetable or tomato juice

By classification, fiber is really considered an indigestible carbohydrate, but it is very different from other carbohydrates—and much lower in calories! It's basically the indigestible part of a plant. It's this inability by the body to break it down that really makes fiber a supernutrient. Fats, proteins, and carbs are like the rabbit from that old fable—they make constant pit stops along the gastrointestinal route and are absorbed into the bloodstream. But fiber is more like the tortoise in that it just keeps going until it hits the colon. It isn't broken down into glucose before it gets to the colon, and often not even there.

However, getting enough fiber into your diet can add roughage in more ways than one. The recommended daily amount (RDA) is 25 grams (for women) to 38 grams (for men), but most of us barely manage 15 grams. If you're unsure if you lean more toward the low-fiber column, you don't have to decipher the nutritional labels. If you answer yes to even one of the following, chances are you need more of the rough stuff in your life:

Do you often feel constipated?

Do you rarely have a daily bowel movement?

Are you often hungry soon after you finish a meal?

The problem is, even if you have the will to eat more fiber, it isn't easy to find a way. The obvious solution—eating six to eight bowls of whole wheat pasta daily—is as unhealthy as it is impractical, not only for dietary reasons, but also because there are two types of nutritional fiber, and you need both.

Insoluble fiber (which doesn't dissolve in water) is like a sponge, expanding as it absorbs liquid in the stomach. It's this extra mass that pushes waste down and out of your system (hello, fiber; goodbye, constipation).

While that may seem like the most important type of fiber to consume, don't forget the other, just as important kind: soluble fiber. In your stomach, soluble fiber binds with liquids to form a gummy gel that makes you feel full as it slows digestion, letting your body absorb more nutrients from the rest of your food. This helps you feel full, reduce cholesterol, stabilize blood sugar levels, and prevent the spike and crash that hits after eating.

Highest-Fiber Fruits and Vegetables

- Apples
- Avocados
- Beans
- Berries (Blueberries, Black-berries, Raspberries, etc.)
- Broccoli*
- Brussels sprouts*
- Cabbage*
- Carrots
- Chick Peas/Garbanzo Beans
- Dried Fruits (Figs, Raisins, Apricots, Dates, etc.)
- Eggplant
- Greens (Collards, Kale, Turnip Greens*)
- Guavas
- Kiwis
- Lima beans
- Mushrooms
- Oranges
- Pears
- Peas (Black-Eyed Peas, Green Peas)
- Peppers
- Potatoes with skin
- Prunes
- Pumpkin, canned
- Rhubarb
- Spinach*
- Sweet Potatoes

* These high-fiber vegetables are also goitrogenic, meaning that they promote thyroid enlargement and can potentially cause or aggravate hypothyroidism. Typically, the risk is highest when these foods are consumed raw, regularly, and in substantial quantity.

Now that fiber is beginning to get the nutritional recognition it deserves, it's often added to yogurt, soy milk, grape juice, those six to eight bowls of whole wheat pasta, and a slew of other non-fiber-related foods. But while those products have their place, they shouldn't be your go-to fiber source. The best way to ingest the stuff is always going to be in its purest form: whole foods.

Which is why a green smoothie is one of the healthiest, as well as most practical, ways of bulking up on fiber. In fact, a green smoothie may be the most effective way to deliver an instant high dose of both kinds of fiber to your body in the shortest amount of time. That's because the indigestible parts of the plant that define fiber are actually fruits, veggies, whole grains, nuts, legumes, and beans—and green smoothies are 100 percent guaranteed to be some variation on this shopping list (see page "Highest-Fiber Fruits and Vegetables" on page 29).

Back to the micronutrients. Those vitamins and minerals are essential to life. They boost the immune system, support normal growth and development, and help cells and organs do their jobs. Without them, we couldn't think or even breathe, much less digest food or walk the dog.

While it seems everything from gum to yogurt is jam-packed with added vitamins and minerals, the reality is that the human body can't really absorb or use these megadoses as efficiently as it does vitamins and minerals from actual whole foods. The even more surprising reality is that most of us are more in danger of getting too many vitamins and minerals than too little. And there's definitely a risk of too much of a good thing even with vitamins and minerals. Ingesting more than the RDA can actually have a toxic bounce back. The breakdown depends on the type of mineral and vitamin.

There are 13 essential vitamins, meaning they are needed for the body to function. While all are organic substances in that they are made by plants or animals, they can be divided into two categories: fat-soluble (A, D, E, and K) and water-soluble (C and the B-complex vitamins such as vitamins B6, B12, niacin, riboflavin, and folate).

It isn't a medical emergency if you ingest too much of the water-soluble vitamins because, as the name says, they need to dissolve in water before your body can absorb them, so your body *can't* store them for later use and will actually flush out the extras. In fact, you need a fresh supply of these vitamins daily.

The problem is with the fat-soluble vitamins. Like the name says, these vitamins dissolve in fat, which means that they can be stored in just about everyone's body. Vitamin A can easily be toxic. Just two to three times the RDA can increase the risks of hip fracture and birth defects. Excessive amounts of vitamin B6 may cause nerve damage.

Minerals, which are inorganic elements that come from soil and water, can also cause problems if overingested. While our bodies need larger amounts of some minerals called macrominerals for optimum functioning, we need only a daily soupçon of trace (so-called because we need only small amounts) minerals like chromium, copper, iodine, iron, selenium, and zinc.

Here is an A to Zinc of the most vital vitamins and minerals, what they do, and the RDA for staying in tip-top shape.

VITAMINS

Vitamin A: Helps eyesight, including night blindness, growth, appetite, and taste.

> *RDA:* 900mcg (Too much can cause birth defects, liver abnormalities, central nervous disorders, and bone density problems.)
>
> *Good Green Smoothie Ingredients:* cod liver oil, carrots, green leafy vegetables, yellow fruits

Vitamin B1 (thiamine): Helps the body's cells convert carbs into energy. It's also essential for the functioning of the heart, muscles, and nervous system.

> *RDA:* 1.2mg
>
> *Good Green Smoothie Ingredients:* dried milk, eggs, legumes, nuts and seeds, peas, whole grains

Vitamin B2 (riboflavin): Helps growth, skin, nails, hair, eyesight, and the breakdown of protein, fat, and carbs.

RDA: 1.6mg

Good Green Smoothie Ingredients: milk, yeast, cheese, green leafy vegetables

Vitamin B3 (niacin): Helps the digestive system, skin, and nerves to function. It's also important for converting food to energy.

RDA: 6mg

Good Green Smoothie Ingredients: dairy products, eggs, legumes, nuts

Vitamin B5 (pantothenic acid): Aids in metabolism, helping the body break down and use food, as well as the production of hormones and cholesterol.

RDA: 5mg

Good Green Smoothie Ingredients: avocado, broccoli, green leafy vegetables, eggs, legumes, milk, mushrooms

Vitamin B6 (pyridoxine): Prevents skin conditions, nerve problems, helps the body absorb protein and carbohydrates.

RDA: 1.3mg (May cause nerve problems in large doses.)

Good Green Smoothie Ingredients: bananas, whole grains, dried beans

Vitamin B7 (biotin): Assists in breaking down and using food.

RDA: 30mcg

Good Green Smoothie Ingredients: chocolate, egg yolks, legumes, milk, nuts

Vitamin B9 (folic acid): Helps in the production of red blood cells and is essential in the first three months of pregnancy to prevent birth defects such as spina bifida, cleft palate, or cleft lip.

RDA: 400mcg, but women planning to conceive should take a daily supplement of 600mcg for the first 12 weeks of pregnancy. Also, this applies only to synthetic folic acid in supplements or fortified foods. There's no upper limit for folic acid from natural sources.

Good Green Smoothie Ingredients: carrots, egg yolks, melon, apricots, pumpkin, avocado, beans, rye and whole wheat, green leafy vegetables

Vitamin B12 (cobalamin): Makes red blood cells and aids in the formation of the nerves.

RDA: 2.4mcg

Good Green Smoothie Ingredients: eggs, milk, cheese

Vitamin C (ascorbic acid): Helps the immune defense system and aids in protection from viruses and bacteria, healing wounds, reducing cholesterol, increasing cell lifespan, and preventing scurvy (in case you're planning a long boat trip).

RDA: 90mg (Large doses can cause diarrhea and nausea and 1000mg or more per day may damage DNA.)

Good Green Smoothie Ingredients: citrus fruits, kiwifruit, berries, tomatoes, cauliflower, potatoes, green leafy vegetables, peppers

Vitamin D: Builds strong bones and teeth.

RDA: 15mcg (The body is a pro at converting natural sources of vitamin D, but too much from supplements can cause poor appetite, nausea and vomiting, and kidney problems.)

Good Green Smoothie Ingredients: cod liver oil, milk, and milk products such as yogurt, dairy-based kefir, and buttermilk

Vitamin E: A powerful antioxidant, it helps fight toxins.

RDA: 15mg (Too much can interfere with blood-thinning meds, and excess of 400IU daily increases risk of heart failure.)

Good Green Smoothie Ingredients: nuts, soy beans, vegetable oil, broccoli, sprouts, spinach, eggs

Vitamin K: Known as the clotting vitamin because without it blood wouldn't clot.

RDA: 120mcg (Too much can interfere with blood-thinning medications.)

Good Green Smoothie Ingredients: green leafy vegetables, Brussels sprouts, broccoli, cauliflower, cabbage, eggs

ESSENTIAL MINERALS: MACROS

Calcium: Good for strong bones and teeth, nerve function, muscle contraction, and blood clotting.

> *RDA:* 1000mg (Excess calcium can be deposited as kidney and gall bladder stones and has been linked to an increased risk for heart attack, headaches, stomach pain, high blood pressure, and diarrhea.)
>
> *Good Green Smoothie Ingredients:* milk, cheese, yogurt, green leafy vegetables

Chloride: Needed to keep the proper balance of body fluids. It's an essential part of digestive (stomach) juices.

> *RDA:* 2.3g (Too much can increase blood pressure and cause a buildup of fluid in people with congestive heart failure, cirrhosis, or kidney disease.)
>
> *Good Green Smoothie Ingredients:* table or sea salt, seaweed, rye grain, tomatoes, lettuce, celery

Magnesium: Aids in converting energy from food, cell repair, building strong bones, teeth, and muscles, regulating body temperature, and 293 other biochemical reactions in the body.

> *RDA:* 400mg (High doses can cause diarrhea.)
>
> *Good Green Smoothie Ingredients:* green leafy vegetables, whole grains, nuts

Phosphorus: Needed to grow and maintain bones and teeth, which store 85 percent of the phosphorus in your body. It's also needed in order for hormones and enzymes to function properly. It's even used to produce DNA and RNA, the genetic molecules in every cell. It also helps in creating, storing, and utilizing energy.

RDA: 700mg (If there's too much phosphorus in your blood, it may leach calcium from your bones, thus making them weak and brittle, which makes them more prone to fractures. Those with chronic kidney disease may need to monitor phosphorus levels closely.)

Good Green Smoothie Ingredients: dairy products like milk and yogurt, nuts, legumes, whole grains

Potassium: Essential to cardiac and tissue health, skeletal contraction, and gastrointestinal function.

RDA: 4,700mg (Abnormally high levels of potassium can lead to potassium toxicity, or hyperkalemia, which can cause muscular weakness, tingling in the extremities, temporary paralysis and, ultimately, death by cardiac arrest due to cardiac arrythmia.)

Good Green Smoothie Ingredients: bananas, prunes, oranges, cantaloupe, avocados, grapes, blackberries, raisins, tomatoes, artichokes, lima beans, acorn squash, carrots, spinach, dairy products, sunflower seeds, almonds

Sodium: In small amounts, sodium is essential for normal nerve and muscle functioning. It's also required for the proper balance of body fluids.

RDA: 2,300mg (It's easy to accidentally overdo since most processed foods are pumped with sodium; too much can result in high blood pressure, heart disease, stroke, and kidney disease.)

Good Green Smoothie Ingredients: sea and table salt, seaweed, celery, Swiss chard

Sulfur: May improve certain health conditions, such as arthritis and liver disorders.

RDA: 900mg

Good Green Smoothie Ingredients: eggs, legumes, whole grains, garlic, onions, Brussels sprouts, cabbage

Slap Me Some Skin

Drop that peeler! The skin is a surprisingly excellent source of vitamins and fiber in many fruits (and vegetables, but we tend to eat many of these with the skin). Much of the insoluble fiber and antioxidants are located in the skin. For example, much of the lemon pith is extremely high in vitamin C and contains vitamin B6 and fiber. And an apple's skin contains anti-cancer properties like polyphenols, as well as pectin, which is known for its ability to lower cholesterol and blood sugar levels.

While you don't have to clean out your bank account to always buy organic (see page 43 for information on when to buy organic), you should always wash all your produce well. This does not mean that you have to stock up on special produce washes or sprays. Studies show that these products aren't any better at removing bacteria or pesticides than water and a little old-fashioned elbow grease. To wash your produce properly, hold the fruit or vegetable under cold running water and gently rub all sides for about 1 minute max.

And the skin isn't the only healthy bit we waste—stalks and cores can also be packed with nutrients. Here, a peel-the-covers-back peek on when to eat the whole fruit and vegetables:

- *Apples:* Skin yes | Seeds no
- *Apricot:* Skin yes | Seed no
- *Avocado:* Skin no | Pit yes with caution
- *Banana:* Peel yes with caution
- *Blackberry:* Seeds yes
- *Cantaloupe and Honeydew:* Rind yes with caution | Seeds yes
- *Cherry:* Skin yes | Pits no
- *Grapes:* Skin yes | Seeds yes
- *Kiwi:* Skin yes | Seeds absolutely
- *Lemon and Lime:* Peel yes | Seeds with caution
- *Mango:* Peel yes with caution | Pit no
- *Orange and Grapefruit:* Peel yes | Seeds yes
- *Peach:* Skin yes | Seed no
- *Pear:* Skin yes | Core no
- *Pineapple:* Top no | Skin yes with caution | Core yes

- *Plum:* Skin yes | Pit no
- *Pumpkin, Butternut, and Other Squashes:* Peel no if raw | Seeds yes
- *Watermelon:* Rind yes | Seeds yes

TRACE MINERALS

Cobalt: A integral part of vitamin B12, cobalt is essential to red blood cell formation and is also helpful to other cells.

> *RDA:* 8mcg, usually fulfilled by ingesting vitamin B12. (Increased intake may affect the thyroid or cause overproduction of red blood cells, thickened blood, and increased activity in the bone marrow.)
> *Good Green Smoothie Ingredients:* milk, legumes, spinach, cabbage, lettuce, beet greens, figs

Copper: Works with iron to form healthy red blood cells.

> *RDA:* 900mcg
> *Good Green Smoothie Ingredients:* nuts, seeds, whole grains

Fluoride: Essential for dental health, helping to prevent cavities.

> *RDA:* 4mg
> *Good Green Smoothie Ingredients:* grape juice (It's worth noting that fluoride is added to most public water systems—but not to bottled water.)

Iodine: Aids thyroid function as well as the cardiovascular, immune, and reproductive systems.

> *RDA:* 150mg (May be toxic to the thyroid if too much is consumed.)
> *Good Green Smoothie Ingredients:* seaweed, iodized salt

Iron: Good for red blood cells, muscle function, white blood cells, and the immune system.

> *RDA:* 8mg (More than 17mg can lead to constipation, vomiting, nausea, and diarrhea, and very high doses can be fatal.)

Good Green Smoothie Ingredients: egg yolks, green leafy vegetables, nuts, whole grains whole wheat

Manganese: The name comes from the Greek word for "magic," which is appropriate as it's known as the antioxidant mineral and has free radical–fighting properties. It aids in food digestion and strengthens bone structure.

RDA: 5mg

Good Green Smoothie Ingredients: asparagus, avocado, bananas, beets, blackberries, cabbage, carrots, cauliflower, coconuts, green peas, honey, whole wheat, lettuce, nuts, peanut butter, pineapple, cheese, spinach, green leafy vegetables

Selenium: Acts like an antioxidant, getting rid of damaging free radicals and reducing the risk of some cancers.

RDA: 55mcg

Good Green Smoothie Ingredients: Brazil nuts, sunflower seeds, milk

Zinc: Helps the immune system and the breakdown of protein, fat, and carbohydrates.

RDA: 11mg (High doses can lead to stomach cramps, nausea, and vomiting.)

Good Green Smoothie Ingredients: milk, brown rice, whole grains

Spoiler Alert

According to those who make a study of these things, we throw out about a fifth of the food in our fridges, or around 470 pounds of food per year per American household. In visual terms, that's about the same size as a cute little pony. In monetary terms, that's around $40 billion worth of meals nationally.

A good portion of what we dump is fruits and vegetables—fruits and vegetables that you had the best intention of making something delicious out of when you bought them, but somehow turned into a slimy brown puddle within a few days of purchasing. While the beautiful thing is that a green smoothie means you can certainly use vegetables and fruits even a little past their best (and some, like bananas, are actually better once they acquire that film noir, bruised look), you may end up losing out on nutrients if the produce is far gone and frankly, why should you use subpar ingredients when the whole point of these smoothies is their nutritional content?

CHAPTER FOUR

The Daily Store

How you choose and store your produce depends on where you're selecting it from.

If you're buying from a farmers' market—or, better yet, growing your own—then you know that everything there is probably as fresh as a teenager with an attitude. But even the most recently picked fruits and vegetables at the supermarket are going to be at least a week (but more likely two weeks) old by the time they land in your shopping cart. So knowing how to buy these items is important.

Shop Right

Surprise, surprise—it may actually be better to hit the freezer section or occasionally, even the canned aisle rather than the fresh produce. Yes, you read that correctly. Here's why: That so-called fresh sugar pea isn't fresh if it's December and you live in a northern region where down coats are a fashion must. Chances are that however appealing it looks, it was picked before it was full-grown (or ripe), which means it has had less time to develop a full spectrum of vitamins and minerals. In addition, during the long haul from farm to fork, fresh fruits and vegetables are exposed to lots of heat and light, which degrade some nutrients, especially delicate vitamins like C and the B vitamin thiamin.

In contrast, that frozen bag of peas is most certainly from the cream of the crop. The peas have been processed (which simply means blanched or steamed in hot water to kill bacteria and slow down food-spoiling enzymes) within a few hours of picking and then flash frozen at their peak ripeness and flavor when vegetables and fruit are usually most nutrient-packed. Look for frozen vegetable and fruit packages marked with a USDA "U.S. Fancy" shield, which identifies produce of the best size, shape, and color; vegetables and fruit with this gold standard also tend to be more nutrient-rich than the lower grades "U.S. No. 1" or "U.S. No. 2." Still, just because something has been given the Ice Age treatment doesn't mean it will last forever. Over many months, nutrients in frozen food will inevitably degrade.

Since the method used for canning produce is somewhat different from frozen, fruits and vegetables in the can may lose some nutrients during the preservation process—primarily vitamin C, which blanches in the high-heat temperature ranges used for canning (although it dissolves in the cooking liquid and can be regained if you don't drain the can prior to use). The other hitch is that salt and sometimes sugar are often added to preserve flavor and prevent spoilage, but there are often low-sodium and -sugar versions available. And, just like the freezing process, vegetables and fruit chosen for canning are picked at peak ripeness and, in some instances, the canned version may be just as healthy and more readily available than frozen; canned tomatoes, pineapple, squash, beans, and pumpkin all tend to keep their healthy bloom. Canned food also has a long shelf life and can be just as good as the day it was packed two or even three years later. But if you see dented or bulging cans, throw them out, as it may be a sign of the rare but deadly food bacteria botulism (it doesn't visibly affect the food, so the can damage is the clue that it may be present).

At the end of the day, the main advantage to buying fresh as opposed to frozen or canned produce in terms of health is that you get the whole fruit and vegetable—skin, seeds, core, and/or stem, which can be jam-packed with antioxidants, vitamins, and nutrients.

What is most definitely not a healthy alternative to fresh veggies and fruit are their dried or juiced sibs.

Although both whole produce and freshly prepared juices have vitamins, minerals and antioxidants, the whole ones are healthier because of their high fiber content. More of a shocker, a glass of orange juice has around the same sugar content as a similar amount of cola.

While dried fruit certainly has an overload of fiber, it's also high on the sugar scales. When food is dehydrated, the natural sugars are concentrated but, because the portion size is smaller, we tend to eat as much if not more. So while a cup of grapes contains about 23 grams of sugar and 104 calories, a cup of raisins weighs in with 100 grams of sugar and 500 calories—about the same as a similar amount of jelly beans!

Get Fresh

To buy the best in produce, take time to give it the onceover.

VEGGIES

Check the stem. This is where that mouthwatering brown rot starts on vegetables like squash, celery, and heads of lettuce. On cucumbers and peppers, the ends will be slightly soft to the touch.

Go green. Lettuce, green beans, and broccoli should be a deep, even green. (In potatoes, though, green can be toxic and should be cut off.)

Pick a nice posy. The tighter the asparagus, broccoli, and cauliflower buds are closed, the fresher they are.

Leaf peep. Broken leaves or yellowed, faded areas mean leafy greens are about to spoil. For those pre-bagged and cut salads that are oh-so-convenient, inspect both sides of the bag to make sure the back of the package looks as good as the front.

Go heavy. Choose lettuce and cabbage heads that are heavy and feel them over for any soft spots that indicate rot.

Skin check. With beans, you want a little give, as a hard shell means it's old and dried out. Root vegetables such as carrots, parsnips, and turnips should feel smooth and firm and on the small side. Overly big tend to have a woody texture.

FRUITS

Look for berries that are plump and have a bright color. Look for strawberries that still have their caps (if they are missing, the berry is too ripe) and look for raspberries and blackberries without a cap (those with a cap are under-ripe).

Plump and firm. Tender fruit like apricots, plums, avocados, and peaches are like Baby Bear's bed from the Goldilocks story—they shouldn't be too hard or too soft but just right at somewhere in between. Try the thumb test: If it leaves a mark, it's too ripe and if it leaves no indentation at all, it's under-ripe. These fruits often ripen over time but just as often simply spoil.

Go heavy. Choose citrus fruit and melons that seem heavy for their size. Don't worry about skin scarring at it does not affect the fruit's taste or nutrients.

Organic or Not Organic? That Is the Question

Is it worth the extra money to splurge on an organic label? It depends.

Organics certainly sound like they fit the healthy, clean philosophy of a green smoothie cleanse, but with a price tag that ranges anywhere from 50 to 100 percent more than nonorganic, filling your eco reusable grocery bag just with organic foods can cause some serious damage to your wallet.

The Dirty Baker's Dozen

Switch to organic for these foods—or to their safe conventionally grown alternatives—and you'll slash your exposure to hormones, pesticides, and antibiotics by 80 percent. If you're craving one of the sweet, crunchy foods here, like bell peppers, try conventional carrots or corn instead. Looking for a safer conventional green? Opt for watercress.

1. **Apples:** Conventional apples have a high fungus and insect risk and may be sprayed up to 16 times with 47 different pesticides. The USDA tests found 98 percent of apples had residues from those sprays. Similar levels are also found in products like apple juice, apple cider, and applesauce. Peeling apples may reduce exposure to pesticide residue, but you're peeling away many of the fruit's most beneficial nutrients. Safe sweet alternatives: watermelons, bananas, and tangerines.

2. **Celery:** Celery is sprayed with organophosphates, which have been linked to ADHD. With no protective skin, they don't wash off. USDA tests have found more than 60 different pesticides on celery. Safe crunchy alternatives: broccoli, radishes, and onions.

3. **Sweet Bell Peppers:** Their soft skin and lack of a protective layer means that these vegetables tend to have almost 50 different kinds of pesticide residue in all of their colorful varieties. Safe sweet alternatives: watermelons, carrots, corn.

4. **Peaches:** Another tree fruit that always makes the dirty dozen list: peaches, with more than 60 pesticides (but far fewer in their canned cousins). Safe sweet alternatives: watermelons, tangerines, oranges, and grapefruit.

5. **Strawberries:** A usual suspect on this list, in part because fungus prompts farmers to spray. Nearly 53 different pesticides have been found on strawberries, though there are fewer when they have been frozen. Safe sweet alternatives: pineapples and kiwis.

6. **Nectarines** (Imported): Domestic nectarines don't test with as much pesticide residue, but overall, 33 pesticides have been detected on nectarines. Safe sweet alternatives: pineapples, papayas, or mangoes.

7. **Grapes** (Imported): Another usual on the "dirty" list, grapes can have more than 30 pesticides. (That cosmopolitan suddenly sounds like a better choice than your usual merlot!) Raisins, not surprisingly, also rank high. Safe sweet alternative: kiwis.

8. **Spinach:** Bugs like spinach more than Popeye does. This popular green leads the leafy green pesticide residue category with nearly 50 different pesticides (frozen had similar levels but canned had fewer). Safe green leafy alternatives: watercress, dandelion greens.

9. **Lettuce:** Another green smoothie mainstay, over 50 different pesticides have been found on virtually all varieties of lettuce. Safe green leafy alternative: watercress.

10. **Cucumber:** Eighty different kinds of pesticide were found on conventional cucumbers. Safe crunchy alternative: asparagus.

11. **Blueberries:** Over 50 pesticides have been detected as residue on blueberries (frozen are slightly less contaminated). Safe sweet alternatives: While cherries and cranberries sound like good, strong antioxidant substitutes, they are often in the gray area between not-quite Dirty Dozen material but not squeaky clean either, so go with bananas instead.

12. **Potatoes:** America's favorite vegetable, spuds have more than 35 pesticide residues. Safe starchy alternative: sweet potatoes.

13. **Collard Greens** (tie): Tests have revealed more than 45 different pesticides on collards. Safe green alternatives: Brussels sprouts, dandelion greens, and cabbage.

13. **Kale** (tie): This green smoothie superfood is actually known as a hardier vegetable that rarely suffers from pests and disease, but it was found to have high amounts of pesticide residue when tested in 2012 and 2013. Safer green alternatives: cabbage, asparagus, dandelion greens, and broccoli.

There are a lot of hidden costs that justify that $$$ price tag. The main one is probably that growing organic requires more work for less results, and this raises the final charge on everything from growing to shipping food. As more big corporations jump on the organic band-wagon, prices will start to drop.

In the meantime, there are a few things you can do to spend less on organics.

First, don't get stuck on the label. There are so many terms and descriptions associated with organic that you practically need a cheat sheet when you go shopping:

- "100% Organic": Product must contain 100 percent organic ingredients.
- "Organic": At least 95 percent of ingredients are organically produced.
- "Made with Organic Ingredients": At least 70 percent of ingredients are organic. The remaining 30 percent must come from the USDA's approved list.
- "Natural" or "All Natural": Does not mean organic. There's no standard definition for this term except with meat and poultry products. (The USDA defines "natural" as not containing any artificial flavoring, colors, chemical preservatives, or synthetic ingredients). The claim isn't verified. The producer or manufacturer alone decides whether to use it.

As to what that organic rating actually means in terms of produce, you can expect that:

- The food has not been genetically modified or irradiated.
- The fertilizer used on the food does not contain sewage sludge or synthetic ingredients.
- Produce has not been contaminated with synthetic chemicals used as pesticides.

However—yes, there is always a however—the best source for these products is local, as there have been more than a few scandals with (usually imported) organic foods that don't meet the requirements or that have actually been adulterated with sometimes even dangerous ingredients.

BANG FOR YOUR BUCK

Now that you know *what* you're shopping for, here's how to save a few dollars:

- Limit your organic shopping to the most potentially toxic foods. The Environmental Working Group analyzes the U.S. Department of Agriculture data about pesticide residue and ranks foods based on how much or little pesticide residue they have into two categories: the Dirty Baker's Dozen (page 44) and the Clean 15 (see page 48).
- Comparison shop: Organic food is showing up in lots of unexpected places, including big-box grocery stores. Many supermarkets are also creating their own organic labels.
- Take advantage of local farmers' markets: Many farmers don't charge a premium.
- Grow your own vegetables and fruits from organic seeds, or pick up fully grown organic plants at farmers' markets or local nurseries: The top-twelve green smoothie ingredients are so fuss-free that even the brownest thumb can grow them from scratch—and no garden is needed as these will all do well in a large container with good drainage:

1. Lettuce
2. Kale
3. Strawberries
4. Fig tree
5. Swiss chard
6. Spinach
7. Radish
8. Beets
9. Basil
10. Parsley
11. Dill
12. Cilantro

The Clean 15

No need to go organic with these foods as they aren't subjected to the worst of the pesticide and hormone drenching. And with proper washing of your produce (which you should do with organics, too), you can get rid of some—but not all—of the pesticide residue.

1. **Onions:** These vegetables have almost no enemies or diseases, making them 99 percent pesticide-free.
2. **Corn:** This one is open to debate. There's little pesticide found on corn (and its husk helps protect the kernels from even that negligible amount), but the low level may be because it's genetically modified to innately deter insects and disease.
3. **Pineapple:** Its spiny skin protects it from pests and pesticide residue.
4. **Avocados:** Their thick skins protect the fruit from pesticide buildup.
5. **Cabbage:** Cabbage does not hold onto so many pesticides because a ton of spraying isn't required to grow it.
6. **Sweet Peas:** Their shells protect them from predators, disease, and pesticide "green washing."
7. **Asparagus:** A hardy perennial vegetable that grows easily in the wild, this vegetable faces fewer threats from pests, therefore less pesticides are used to cultivate it.
8. **Mango:** Another fruit whose thick skin helps to protect it from pesticides.
9. **Eggplant:** Its thick skin may be what keeps natural predators, disease, and the effects of the pesticide sprayers away.
10. **Kiwi:** Its fuzzy skin acts as a barrier to pesticides.
11. **Cantaloupe:** With that rind, this melon has a natural defense against the onslaught of any chemical.
12. **Sweet Potato:** Considered a superfood, sweet potato is packed with vitamin A and beta-carotene, and is also pesticide-free.
13. **Grapefruit:** The peel isn't eaten, and that's where the pesticide stays.
14. **Watermelon:** Pesticide residue stays on the thick rind, but rinse before cutting.
15. **Mushrooms:** With no known predators, this fungus stays safe from pesticides.

Storing Up

Obviously, it helps if you start blending—or at least chopping and freezing to blend later—your produce as soon as you can. But if you don't have the time, you should still make the effort to do a little prep beyond opening the fridge and tossing your shopping bag onto the emptiest shelf.

Prep Tip I: Some fruits emit ethylene, an odorless, colorless gas that accelerates ripening and, if it's ultraresponsive, spoilage in some fruits and vegetables. (If you want to speed-ripen some fruits, try this ethylene-trapping science experiment: Put berry fruits in a closed paper bag with a ripe banana). Treat your produce like your laundry and separate your ethylene-prone from your ethylene-sensitive produce (or invest in a product that absorbs the ethylene):

High-Ethylene Produce That Should Be Refrigerated

Apples

Apricots

Cantaloupes

Figs

Honeydew melons

High-Octane Produce That Shouldn't Be Refrigerated

Avocados

Bananas, unripe

Nectarines

Peaches

Pears

Plums

Tomatoes

Ethylene Sensitive (see Prep Tip 1 for Storage)

Bananas, ripe

Broccoli

Brussels sprouts

Cabbage

Carrots

Cauliflower

Cucumbers

Eggplant

Lettuce and other leafy greens

Squash

Parsley

Sweet potatoes

Peas

Watermelons

Peppers

Prep Tip 2: Potatoes, sweet potatoes, onions, garlic, and winter squash such as pumpkin and butternut fare better out of the moist fridge. Instead, separate each vegetable group in its own well-ventilated container (baskets work well) and store in a cool, dark place.

Prep Tip 3: Wrap greens like lettuce, kale, and spinach in a slightly moistened paper towel, put in a loosely closed bag, and store in the vegetable crisper/drawer. Change the paper towel daily.

Prep Tip 4: One bad apple—or any fruit or vegetable—really can spoil the whole bunch. Mold multiplies like Einstein doing math and contaminates everything nearby, so toss any spoiled produce immediately. For longer life, keep your produce whole; don't even rip the stem out of an apple until you eat it. As soon as you start pulling things apart, you break the cells and microorganisms start to grow.

Prep Tip 5: Honor your produce's origins. The rule of thumb is if it comes from a tropical or warm climate, keep it out of the cold. Pineapple, tomatoes, bananas, and mangoes are all hot produce. Store them on the counter, not in the fridge. Once they're fully ripe, you can refrigerate them to help them last.

Prep Tip 6: Keep things loose. Produce needs to breathe. The worst thing to do is seal fruits and vegetables in an airtight bag as you'll "suffocate" them and speed up decay.

Prep Tip 7: Dunk it. Herb stalks stay fresh when their feet are kept wet and their heads dry. Fill a glass halfway with water and put the herbs in stem-first. Loosely cover the whole shebang with one of those plastic produce bags from the supermarket. Change the water every few days.

When to Eat It

Some types of produce are like houseguests and shouldn't hang around for more than a few days. Others are hardy and can literally keep for as long as a year. Use this timeline to know what to eat when:

Spoiler Alert: Eat within one to three days once ripe

Artichokes	Dill
Asparagus	Green beans
Avocados	Mushrooms
Bananas	Mustard greens
Basil	Strawberries
Cherries	Watercress
Corn	

Spoiler Alert: Eat within three to five days once ripe

Arugula	Mesclun
Grapes	Zucchini
Lettuce	

Spoiler Alert: Eat within one week once ripe

Apricots	Oregano
Bell peppers	Parsley
Blueberries	Peaches
Broccoli	Pears
Cauliflower	Pineapples
Celery	Plums
Cucumbers	Spinach
Eggplant	Tomatoes
Mint	Watermelons

Spoiler Alert: Eat within one to three months once ripe

Apples

Beets

Brussels sprouts

Cabbage

Carrots

Grapefruits

Leeks

Lemons

Limes

Oranges

Potatoes

Spoiler Alert: Eat within six months to a year once ripe

Garlic

Onions

Winter squash

Chew on This

Q: When is a fruit not a fruit? A: When it's a vegetable.

These are vegetables:

- Artichoke
- Broccoli
- Carrots
- Cauliflower
- Potato
- Radish
- Rhubarb

And the following are—surprise!—fruits:

- Avocado
- Bell Pepper
- Cucumber
- Eggplant
- Nuts (including coconuts)
- Okra
- Squash
- Tomato*

And these are what can, for now, be listed very unscientifically under "Other":

- Banana (although it's a fruit, the plant it's grown from is classified as an herb)
- Bean (legume)
- Corn (grain)
- Lentil (legume)
- Peanut (legume)
- Peas (legume)
- Mushroom (fungus)

Fruits are assumed to be sweet and vegetables are assumed to be the mostly green stuff that kids don't like. But it isn't that simple. The difference between the two however, lies in classification, not taste buds.

The botanical definition for a fruit is that it is the mature ovary of a flower, containing the seed.

Translation: Do you eat the seeds? If the answer is yes, it's a fruit. Vegetables—such as beets, carrots, celery, kale, lettuce, and spinach—may start from seed but the seed isn't a part of what we eat of these plants. So they are categorized as vegetables.

In 1983, the United States Supreme Court decided unanimously that a tomato is a vegetable, even though it's a botanical fruit.

CHAPTER FIVE

It's Easy Drinking Green

Many of us seem to have a complicated relationship with vegetables. Even if you somehow missed one of the news reports that come out practically daily touting how a diet rich in vegetables can improve health, you probably heard it from your parents or learned it back when you were at school or have been given the vegetable riot act by your doctor or read/saw/listened to Dr. Oz or caught it on a late night TV celebrity interview. But knowing does not necessarily mean doing. Too often, our best intentions end up decomposing in the produce drawer into something that could be used as a prop in *The Swamp Thing* when life becomes too busy to think about peeling and dicing.

That is because we want health but we also want taste, convenience, and low cost. While you can just grab an apple on the run, what are you going to do with a bag full of kale?

Hello, green smoothie! They are easy to make, a simple way to use up leftover or I-know-I-bought-it-but-what-the-heck-do-I-do-with-it veggies, and a quick means of getting all of those crucial daily servings of vegetables on the go.

Dark, green leafy vegetables are probably the vegetables we struggle to eat the most of (and therefore the vegetable most likely to be wilting in your fridge). But they are also amazing sources of disease-fighting antioxidants, vitamins, minerals, phytonutrients, fiber, and healthy omega-3 fats. Plus they are practically carb-free and, although filling and slow for the body to digest, ultra-low in calories, making them (in diner menu–parlance) a "dieter's delight."

Because greens have very few carbohydrates and a lot of fiber, they take the body a long time to digest. If you're on a diet, leafy greens can be your best friend; they fill you up, but they have very few calories and no fat. In fact, most greens have such little impact on blood glucose that many low-carb diets consider them "free foods."

The nutritional profile of a typical green leafy vegetable would include most if not all of the following:

Vitamin A
- maintaining normal reproduction
- good vision
- formation and maintenance of healthy skin, teeth, and soft tissues of the body
- immune function (has antioxidant properties)
- Vitamin B6
- breaking down, using, and reforming the building blocks of proteins

Vitamin C
- full of antioxidants
- slows bone loss
- helps the body make collagen, a major component of cartilage that aids in joint flexibility
- protects against arthritis
- helps keep skin and hair photo-worthy
- aids in the absorption of iron and copper

- helps fight infection
- helps regenerate and stabilize other vitamins such as vitamin E or folate

Vitamin E
- helps to keep skin healthy
- protects skin from the sun's damaging rays
- may help reduce risk of cataracts and macular degeneration
- acts as an antioxidant, particularly for fats
- keeps the heart, circulation, skin, and nervous system in good condition

Vitamin K
- regulates blood clotting
- helps protect bones from osteoporosis
- may help prevent and possibly even reduce atherosclerosis by reducing calcium in arterial plaques
- may be a key regulator of inflammation, and may help protect us from inflammatory diseases, including arthritis
- may help prevent diabetes

Beta-carotene
- contributes to the growth and repair of the body's tissues
- protects skin against sun damage
- converts to vitamin A in the body (food is the best and safest way to get your daily fix of this vitamin, since the extremely high doses of vitamin A in supplements can be toxic and lead to bone, liver, and neural disorders, as well as birth defects)

Calcium
- keeps teeth and bones strong
- reduces overall risk for osteoporosis

- aids muscle and nerve function
- helps with blood-pressure management

Chlorophyll
- may aid in carrying oxygen in blood

Folate
- protects against memory loss
- contributes to the production of serotonin and may therefore help ward off depression and improve mood
- breaking down and using the building blocks of proteins to keep the body functioning optimally
- aids the processes of tissue growth and cell function
- maintains good heart health
- prevents neural tube defects in newborns

Insoluble Fiber
- helps digestion
- lowers cholesterol and triglycerides
- may help to prevent ulcers, particularly duodenal ulcers, diabetes, heart disease, and some gastric/colon-related cancers

Iron
- helps to transport oxygen throughout the body, protecting women especially from anemia
- helps keep cells, skin, hair, and nails healthy

Lutein and Zeaxanthin
- antioxidants that help reduce risk of cataracts and macular degeneration

Magnesium
- aids the functioning of more than 300 enzyme systems
- increases energy production

- regulates potassium levels
- helps with the use of calcium
- helps maintain healthy bones
- helpful mineral for those with type-2 diabetes

Potassium

- helps with nerve impulses
- helps with muscle contraction
- regulates blood pressure
- helps create enzymes needed for digestion

Quercetin

- antioxidant
- acts as an anti-inflammatory
- may protect against cancer cell growth
- blocks substances involved in allergies
- causes a decrease in the release of interleukin-6, which may help with appetite suppression

No wonder dark, green leafy vegetables are, calorie for calorie, the nutritional powerhouses of any green smoothie. You can chuck other vegetables in the blender too (see Add-Ins, page 211), but the bulk of your greens should come from this list:

Arugula	Lamb's-quarters
Bok choy	Mustard greens
Broccoli rabe	Parsley
Collard greens	Red and green leaf lettuce
Escarole	Romaine lettuce
Dandelion greens	Spinach
Frisee lettuce	Sprouts
Green cabbage	
Kale	

Have It Your Way

Some of the leafy vegetables in green smoothies can be an acquired taste, which you'll almost definitely acquire the more you drink them. But in the meantime, work within your flavor comfort zone. You can add a handful of stronger-tasting stuff each time and slowly increase the ratio.

Best for Newbies—If you're just starting to blend, try these milder-tasting greens:

- Bok choy
- Carrot greens
- Celery greens
- Escarole
- Frisee lettuce
- Parsley
- Red and green leaf lettuce
- Spinach
- Swiss chard

Better for Those in the Know—These heartier, sometimes peppery greens are just the ticket when you're ready to step up your smoothie game:

- Arugula
- Beet greens
- Broccoli Rabe
- Dandelion greens
- Lamb's-quarters
- Green cabbage
- Mustard greens
- Romaine lettuce
- Tatsoi
- Turnip greens
- Watercress

Ideal for the Blending Whiz—The stronger flavors and textures of these greens let you show your Greenie chops:

- Collard greens
- Kale

Swiss chard

Tatsoi

Watercress

You can be a purist and use one type of green per smoothie or you can mix 'n' match.

Either way, it's a good idea to jumble things up regularly or, as the Greenies say, rotate your greens on at least a weekly basis. First, this will make sure you get the full nutritional benefits of all of the greens. Second, it might be easy to have a go-to tried-and-true green that you always use, but it's going to get gastronomically boring mighty fast.

Last, moderation is always the key word when it comes to diet. Too much of anything—even a good thing—can have a backlash effect, and an overabundance of minerals, vitamins, and compounds in dark, leafy greens are no different. A couple of cups daily of these greens is probably fine, but drink a few smoothies a day and you can easily absorb a pound of leaves, which might become a problem. For instance, spinach and collards are high in oxalic acid, which is generally safe but doesn't play well with pre-existing conditions, such as for those who are prone to kidney stones or rheumatoid arthritis.

Swap greens from different family gene pools to ensure you stay in the pink:

Cruciferae

Arugula

Bok choy

Broccoli rabe

Collard greens

Green cabbage

Kale

Mustard greens

Radish greens

Tatsoi

Turnip greens

Watercress

Amaranthaceae

Beet greens

Lamb's-quarters

Spinach

Swiss chard

Asteraceae

Escarole

Dandelion greens

Frisee lettuce

Red and green leaf lettuce

Romaine lettuce

Apiaceae

Carrot greens

Celery greens

Parsley

Drink Your Compost!

Beets, carrots, radishes, and turnips often show up in supermarkets with no tops attached at all, so it's easy to overlook these greens as potential smoothie ingredients. Even if you do buy your veggies fully loaded, you probably toss their tops when preparing a meal. Don't. Instead, pitch these surprising "spare parts" into your smoothie:

Strawberry Tops: Think of all the time you'll save on slicing your berries. Strawberry greens aren't only edible, they're like any green and full of vitamins and minerals.

Carrot Greens: Carrots are in the parsley family, so their tops closely resemble the herb. There's some controversy over whether they are toxic, but research has established that the danger is probably a result of pesticides.

Radish Greens: You don't have to be a radish lover to like their greens. Rather than bitter or peppery, their flavor is mild and tastes a lot like beet roots or turnips.

Celery Greens: Just think of them as the head and hair of the celery stalk with exactly the same nutritional value—but with a much more delicate flavor.

Beet Greens: Unlike the beets themselves, which have a strong, earthy tang, the greens taste a lot like Swiss chard and can be used in place of that vegetable or spinach in smoothie recipes.

Turnip Greens: These are similar to beet greens, with a dollop more flavor.

Cauliflower Leaves: Unsurprisingly, since they are in the same Brassica family, they have a taste similar to cabbage.

See page 43 for information on when to buy organic.

CHAPTER SIX

Accessorize Your Green Smoothie

You really can't make a green smoothie any simpler: Throw some leafy greens, fruit, and water in a blender, whir, and presto! You've made yourself one of the most nutrient-dense drinks in the world with off-the-chart numbers for a cocktail of vitamins, minerals, and antioxidants.

However, you can also make a green smoothie more complicated. There are oodles of things you can add to your drink to make it sweeter, spicier, or transform it into an energy drink or a dinner replacement. A walk down any supermarket aisle will give you plenty of ideas to come up with your own flavor combos. Millions of dollars have been invested in product research to put together the perfect blend of flavors, so go ahead and piggyback off of their efforts. Or choose something from the list below. With the exception of the sweeteners, all of these extra add-ins qualify as "superfoods" in that the have a strong concentration of phytonutrients, vitamins, minerals, and enzymes that can help to prevent or even reverse one or more chronic, debilitating, and often deadly diseases and are high in good fats and protein. It won't be long before you've earned your Iron Chef title and are powering up your green smoothie with a spice combo to make it taste like apple pie.

But initially, the phrase to remember is: Less is more. In other words, start adding single ingredients, use a smaller amount than you think you need, and always blend and taste after each addition.

Drink Your Vegetables

You have the green leafy kind down cold, but there's a world of vegetables out there just ready for blending. Back to that USDA recommendation of 9 cups daily. It isn't just a matter of eating more fruits and vegetables; consuming a variety of different-colored produce is important as well.

Different hues in fruits and vegetables tend to correspond to different combinations of nutrients and other phytochemicals, each with its own assortment of health benefits. So the more colors in your green smoothie, the more you reap the healthy benefits. The trick to eating by color is to include the skins (see Slap Me Some Skin, page 36), the richest sources of protective phytonutrients, along with the paler flesh.

Here is the color of a healthy diet:

Red: Tomatoes, red onions, radishes, red bell peppers, radicchio, rhubarb, red potatoes. *Colorcharge*: Lycopene, a potent scavenger of gene-damaging free radicals that seems to protect against prostate cancer as well as heart and lung disease. Lycopene may help lower bad cholesterol levels. Anthocyanin, which is a healthy heart antioxidant.

Red/Purple: Beets, red cabbage, red peppers. *Colorcharge*: Anthocyanins and polyphenols, which are believed to delay cellular aging, aid brain function, and help the heart by blocking the formation of blood clots.

Blue/Purple: Eggplant, purple cabbage, purple beans, purple potatoes, purple asparagus, purple carrots, purple Belgian endive. *Colorcharge*: Ellagic acid, an anti-aging compound that may guard against cancer.

Orange: Carrots, sweet potatoes, winter squash, orange cauliflower, orange bell peppers. *Colorcharge*: The cancer-fighter alpha carotene, along with beta-carotene, which may help boost the immune system, maintain healthy skin and bones, and keep eyesight healthy, and beta cryptothanxin, which supports intracellular communication and may help prevent heart disease.

Yellow: Carrots, corn, yellow/golden beets, yellow peppers, yellow pumpkins, yellow potatoes, rutabagas, yellow summer squash, yellow sweet potatoes, yams. *Colorcharge*: Vitamin C, which strengthens the immune system.

Green/Pale Green: Broccoli, Brussels sprouts, green peas, avocados, green cauliflower, asparagus, artichokes, tomatillos, zucchini, green beans, green peppers, leeks, okra, cucumber, fava beans, lima beans, fennel, soy beans. *Colorcharge*: Cancer-blocking chemicals like sulforaphane, isocyanate, and indoles, which inhibit the action of carcinogens; lutein and zeaxanthin, which have been linked to a reduced risk of cataracts and age-related macular degeneration; chlorophyll, which is a natural blood purifier and an anti-inflammatory.

White/Tan: Garlic, onions, leeks, white asparagus, white carrots, daikon, white radishes, potatoes, turnips, jicama, cauliflower, mushrooms, parsnips, white corn, Jerusalem artichokes, kohlrabi, bean sprouts, broad beans, plantains, ginger root. *Colorcharge*: Allicin, a compound in onions and garlic, which may inhibit tumor growth. Some white foods also contain flavonoids, which help reduce risk of heart disease and some cancers.

Sow Some Seeds

It isn't that surprising that seeds are literally, well, seeded with nutrients. After all, the seed is like the plant's egg, the growing and feeding station for the future plant. So it's going to be a veritable buffet bar of vitamins, minerals, and nourishing compounds. They rank in the top five of plant sources of iron and zinc.

Some seeds are also incredibly high in protein. And not just the garden or common variety of proteins found in vegetables and fruit, but what is known as "complete proteins." In order to build muscle, skin, and other important parts of the body, you need 21 amino acids, nine of which are considered "essential" because you can't make them on your own; you have to get them through food. A complete protein, like animal meat, contains all nine of those essential amino acids, while an incomplete protein, like grains or legumes, is deficient in one or more of them. But some seeds, like hemp and amaranth, are unique in that they have as much protein as meat does.

However, seeds are also high in fat (albeit the good kind of fat that helps to minimize the accumulation of LDL cholesterol) and calories, so it's best to use them in small doses—and quickly, as the fat can cause them to spoil easily (store in the refrigerator or freezer). Luckily, a little is all you need—one little tablespoon of pumpkin seeds contains almost twice as much iron as an ounce of skinless chicken breast. And they provide more fiber per ounce than nuts and are also good sources of protein.

Here are the top seeds:

Amaranth (*58 calories and 2 grams of fat per ¼ cup*) You have probably never heard of amaranth, but you should definitely be eating it. While the entire plant can be broken down for eating, the tiny seeds—which are often called pseudo-grains because they're not true cereal grains—are, like hemp seeds, a complete protein. The size of poppy seeds, they have a nutty taste and are also high in fiber, calcium, iron, potassium, phosphorus, and vitamins A and C.

Raw Cacao/Cocoa Powder (*260 calories and 13 grams of fat per ¼ cup*) Made from the seed of the tree, cacao/cocoa is chocolate in raw form, before fat, sugar, and other "sweeteners" are added so it adds an instant yum factor to your green smoothie. If you needed another excuse to eat chocolate guilt-free, it also contains over 300 compounds including protein, fat, carbohydrates, fiber, iron, zinc, copper, calcium, magnesium, and sulfur, as well as the feel-good chemicals phenylethylamine (PEA) and anandamide.

Chia Seeds *(137 calories and 12 grams of fat per ¼ cup)* Yes, this is the same stuff as the Chia Pet of infomercial fame, but it's so much more than just easy-to-grow grass. Extremely tiny, yet extremely potent, the seeds are actually packed full of omega-3 fatty acids, carbohydrates, protein, antioxidants, and even calcium. They have more fiber, ounce for ounce, than wheat germ. Because they have a mild, nutty flavor, chia seeds are easy to add to a variety of foods and drinks. Be warned—when mixed with liquid, they turn your green smoothie into a green gel that can be difficult to slurp through a straw but supposedly creates a type of weight-loss pudding that can help control hunger.

Flaxseed *(224 calories and 18 grams of fat per ¼ cup)* Rich in omega-3 fatty acids, dietary fiber, and lignans (beneficial plant compounds), flaxseeds may lower your risk of heart disease, cancer, stroke, and diabetes. Flaxseeds are best ground before eating for better absorption of the nutrients. (You can easily crush them yourself in an electric coffee grinder.)

Hemp Seeds *(162 calories and 18 grams of fat per ¼ cup)* More commonly associated with an illicit drug, hemp is actually an excellent source of essential fatty acids, fiber, and contains all nine essential amino acids, making the seeds a complete protein source.

Pumpkin Seeds *(72 calories and 3 grams of fat per ¼ cup)* Slightly sweet and nutty with a chewy texture, pumpkin seeds are lower in fat than other seeds and high in essential minerals like iron, magnesium, and potassium. They rank high in the immunity-boosting carotenoid antioxidants, omega-3 fatty acids, and zinc—two important nutrients that may play a role in warding off inflammation, arthritis, and osteoporosis—as well as protective compounds called phytosterols, which aid in keeping stable levels of cholesterol and enhancing immune response, as well as providing cancer-fighting benefits.

Quinoa (*68 calories and 2 grams of fat per ¼ cup*) It may often be lumped with grains, but it's actually a seed. No matter what its classification, this protein source contains a complete set of branch-chain and essential amino acids, making it a tissue- and muscle-building powerhouse.

Sesame Seeds (*182 calories and 15 grams of fat per ¼ cup*) Sesame seeds aren't just for hamburger buns. These powerhouse seeds provide calcium, iron, magnesium, phosphorus, zinc, B and E vitamins, and dietary fiber. Due to their antioxidants, they may help lower inflammation and cholesterol, inhibit cancer cell growth, improve brain health, and prevent arthritis, asthma, migraine headaches, menopause, osteoporosis, and PMS. Open sesame!

Sunflower Seeds (*207 calories and 19 grams of fat per ¼ cup*) Not just for the birds, these seeds are a mine of minerals like iron, folate, selenium, magnesium, and zinc, and are also rich in protein and dietary fiber. In fact, sunflower seeds are the best whole-food source of vitamin E. They're also packed with four times more antioxidants than that superfood favorite blueberries and are full of good fats.

Strengthen the Proteins

Proteins are the building blocks of life. Every cell in the human body contains the stuff. It's a major part of the skin, muscles, organs, and glands. You need protein in your diet to help your body maintain, repair, and make new cells.

If you eat dairy and meat, you're probably digesting all of the protein you need in your daily diet. However, if you're a vegan or vegetarian, you may be on the "low end" protein-wise, which may cause physical and mental fatigue. Like anything, moderation is the key; it's possible to have too much protein, which can put a strain on the kidneys and, if your protein source is meat, contribute to high cholesterol levels or other diseases such as gout. Two to three servings of protein-rich food (like lean meat, beans, nuts, cheese, and eggs) will meet the daily needs of most adults. Another way to do the math is to calculate that you need 0.5 to 0.75 grams of protein daily for every pound of body weight.

These foods will instantly power up the protein level of your green smoothie, transforming it into a whole meal:

Protein Powders: Basic protein powders are made of whey, soy, hemp, rice, eggs, casein (the type of protein usually found in dairy foods), or fish. However—and this is a significant caveat—there's little or no uniformity among products, the labels are confusing (the dose recommended on the bottle may be much higher than the dose recommended by your doctor), and the powders are also minimally regulated, with a majority going untested by the Food and Drug Administration. Doctors and nutritionists agree that people who eat a normal diet generally don't need protein-heavy supplements, even if they are gym rats, and that powders may cause more problems than power in the long run, including stomach upset and muscle cramps.

If you do decide to take a powder, know that a pinch of this stuff will go a long way. Some have 80 grams of protein per serving. To put that in perspective, the body only needs between 10 and 14 additional grams of protein per day to build a pound of muscle.

There are also high-quality plant-based protein powders on the market with straightforward ingredient lists, but they can be expensive. Flavors vary from strong and chemical to nutty to none at all. See Make It, Don't Buy It (page 82) for recipes for your own powder.

Tofu: Tofu will make your green smoothie milkshake creamy delicious—without the sugar and fat and no discernible added flavor. A soybean product made from the pressed curds of soy milk, it's light and easily digestible, and a fine source of vegetarian protein. A half-cup of tofu delivers 10 grams of protein for only 88 calories (about half as much protein but 45 fewer calories than the same amount of roasted, skinless chicken), magnesium, iron and zinc (both needed for cell-growth and immunity building), bone-strengthening calcium, omega-3 fatty acids, selenium, and copper, yet tofu is low in fat and very low in saturated fat. Some studies show it can lower cholesterol and may even help prevent certain types of cancers.

DAIRY PRODUCTS

With the exception of powdered milk, which is tasteless, dairy products add a strong and sometimes grainy tang to smoothies. A dollop of dried powdered milk, buttermilk (page 88), yogurt (page 86), kefir (page 84), which is a dairy drink made from fermenting kefir grains in milk or creamy cheeses like cottage (page 88), goat milk, or ricotta (page 87) will make your smoothie extra thick and creamy and add a healthy dose of casein. Casein is a slower-digesting protein that will continue to feed your muscles hours after your last sip. Keep the calorie count low by aiming for low or no fat and, in the case of cottage cheese, low sodium. Greek yogurt (page 87) will have twice the protein of regular yogurt, while kefir is similar to yogurt in that they are both probiotic, containing heaps of beneficial bacteria. The difference is while yogurt helps keep the digestive system clean and provides food for the friendly bacteria that live there, kefir colonizes the intestinal tract, helping the body become more efficient in resisting such pathogens as E. coli and intestinal parasites.

EGGS

The incredible edible egg is a small complete package of protein, supplying all of the essential amino acids. When uncooked, they also supply a basket of vitamins and minerals, including retinol (vitamin A), riboflavin (vitamin B2), folic acid, vitamins B6 and 12, choline, calcium, iron, phosphorus, potassium, and even CoQ10. However, while raw is the easiest way to add an egg to a smoothie, it isn't necessarily the healthiest. Raw eggs are associated with salmonella, although contamination is rare—less than 1 in 20,000 eggs—and nearly 80 billion eggs are produced in the United States each year. If you already had your protein today, then you have probably already figured out that that means as many as 400,000 eggs could test positive for salmonella. So unless you're 1,000 percent confident of your egg source (and if you're not, stop eating the raw cookie dough when you bake!), opt for the powdered kind (available as powdered whites, yolks, and whole eggs), usually found in the baking section (the whites might be called "meringue powder"). These dehydrated eggs have the same nutritional content as their raw flock without the potential contamination. Eggs will add no discernible flavor to your smoothies.

Green Powder

The bottom line is that no one really needs to add these pulverized multivitamins to their green smoothies. The whole idea of the drink is to give you all of your vitamins and minerals in one long, tasty slurp. While your body is mostly going to flush out any extra water-soluble vitamins (vitamins C and B complex) with no harm done, there are inherent risks in shoring up fat-soluble vitamins through supplements—overdoses of vitamin A can reduce bone-mineral density, leading to osteoporosis, cause bone and joint pain, liver and nerve abnormalities, hair loss, blurred vision, and, if taken by pregnant women, birth defects. An excess of vitamin D can cause nausea, vomiting, poor appetite, constipation, weakness, and can raise the level of calcium in the blood, which can lead to mental confusion and abnormal heart rhythms. Too much vitamin E may actually have a reverse effect and increase the risk for heart failure, especially in people with cardiovascular disease. The anti-coagulant properties of vitamin K means overloading may increase the risk for bleeding problems.

That said, certain supplemental powders are safe to put in to your smoothie because they contain some of the more elusive vitamins and minerals:

Camu Powder: Made from camu berries, this powder is packed with more vitamin C than any orange you'll ever eat. It has a strong tart taste, so all you need is 1 teaspoon.

Matcha or Maca Green Tea Powder: Because the whole tea leaf is ingested, as opposed to just the steeped water in the case of green teas served hot, a small scoop of this slightly sweet powder will deliver a much higher potency of catechin flavenoids, chlorophyll, and antioxidants (by weight, matcha contains more antioxidants than blueberries, pomegranates, orange juice, and spinach).

Spirulina Powder: Unfortunately, this powder tastes a lot like what it is—blue-green pond algae. However, a couple of tablespoons is the equivalent of eating a steak's worth of protein and omega-3 fatty acids without the cholesterol.

Chlorella Powder: Another "delicious" algae, chlorella—whose name comes from its practically obscene amounts of chlorophyll—is packed not only with this cleansing nutrient (nearly ten times that of similar greens like wheat grass, barley, and alfalfa), but also protein, iron, calcium, magnesium, potassium, vitamin A, vitamin B12, vitamin C, and vitamin E.

Things to Chew On

Add texture to your smoothie and pump up the super power with these added ingredients. Unlike Hollywood celebrities and boy bands, all of these deserve their hype.

Goji Berries: A half-cup of these sweet Asian berries will add a handful of antioxidants, amino acids, and more than 20 vitamins and minerals. Soak in water first to soften them and make blending easier.

Açaí Berries: Pronounced "uh-sigh-ee," these Brazilian beauties are loaded with antioxidants that boost your body's energy and ability to focus, along with protein and fiber that will keep you feeling full. Most easily found in powder form, their tart, slightly bitter taste works well sweet or savory smoothies. All you need is a tablespoon to reap the health benefits.

Whole Grains: Think wheat (germ, cracked, or berries), buckwheat, millet, spelt, oats, barley, brown rice, faro, and rye. Their high fiber content provides a bevy of protection against heart disease, cancer, and diabetes. It also thickens up your smoothie quickly, so use sparingly or you may end up with a drink as thick and undrinkable as wet cement. Because of their unsaturated fat content, whole grains can turn rancid easily, so store in the fridge or freezer to maintain freshness.

Nuts and Nut Butters

You would have to be nuts to miss out on the healthy fat power players. Just a handful ups the protein and fiber totals while adding taste and texture to your smoothie. See Make It, Don't Buy It (page 82) for recipes to make your own. Here's the breakdown of the healthiest nuts:

Almonds *(160 calories and 14 grams of fat per 1 ounce)* Those high fat numbers are all good because almonds have nearly nine times more monounsaturated healthy fat than dangerous saturated fat, with plenty of protein, fiber, calcium, vitamin E, and iron thrown in. A handful a day—about 23 almonds—can actually help lower LDL cholesterol levels and fight inflammation.

Walnuts *(190 calories and 18 grams of fat per 1 ounce)* Walnuts stand out for their heart-healthy omega-3 fatty acid content and abundance of polyunsaturated fat, which may protect against type-2 diabetes.

Pistachios: *(160 calories and 13 grams of fat per 1 ounce)* Thought to have the highest level of fiber and LDL-cholesterol-lowering plant sterols, pistachios are nearly as high in monounsaturated fat as almonds and a are rich source of potassium and carotenoids, including beta carotene and lutein. Use the undyed kind.

Peanuts *(170 calories and 14 grams of fat per 1 ounce)* OK, so they are really a legume, but peanuts are commonly lumped with nuts and are another nutty choice for lowering cholesterol levels and triglycerides, decreasing heart disease risk. These "fake" nuts also provide more protein (7 grams per serving) than the real kinds.

Hazelnuts *(180 calories and 17 grams of fat per 1 ounce)* In addition to their high content of vitamin E, manganese, and fiber, hazelnuts rank number one among tree nuts in folate content, decreasing the risk of birth defects, cardiovascular disease, and depression. They also have the highest content of any tree nut of the heart-healthy compound proanthocyanidin, known for contributing astringent flavor to foods and reducing the risk of blood clotting and urinary tract infections.

Pecans *(200 calories and 20 grams of fat per 1 ounce)* One of the most antioxidant-rich nuts, pecans are also high in flavonoids and plant sterols, natural compounds that help lower cholesterol.

Spice It Up

Spices and herbs are much more than fat- and sugar-free flavor boosters. They are also bursting with antioxidants and metabolic and anti-inflammatory properties (inflammation has been identified as a precursor to many chronic diseases, such as heart disease, allergies, and Alzheimer's). Apparently, good things do come in small packages.

While many spices and herbs have some beneficial effects, these are the ones to add a dash of in your green smoothie:

Cinnamon: One teaspoon contains the same antioxidant level as a half-cup of blueberries. It's also rich in polyphenols, which can act like insulin and help regulate blood sugar levels. However, the stuff in your spice rack is more likely an impostor known as cassia. True cinnamon, often labeled "Ceylon cinnamon," has higher levels of antioxidants.

Chile/Dried Red Peppers: People have been cooking with chile peppers for almost 10,000 years. Japanese karate athletes eat chile to strengthen their willpower, and African farmers use it to keep elephants away from their crops. The magic ingredient is capsaicin, which acts as a pain reliever for headaches, arthritis, and other chronic pain problems by inhibiting the release of P-protein, which in turn interrupts the transmission of constant pain signals to the brain. Capsaicin has also been linked to the release of bliss-out endorphins and the regulation of blood sugar. Chiles are also a diet food, helping to boost metabolism, increase fullness, and possibly stimulate fat burning. Even if fiery foods aren't to your taste, don't skip on this spice. As little as a healthy pinch can reap the good effects. If you do accidentally overload, don't gulp water; have some milk instead. Capsaicin isn't water-soluble, but the caseins in dairy products seem to put up a firewall against chile pepper heat.

Ginger: Most potent in root form, ginger is a digestive aid, helping to sooth nausea, speed food through the digestive tract, and protect against gastric ulcers. It may also help with pain, including menstrual cramps, muscle pain, and migraines, and act as a COX-2 inhibitor (a form of nonsteroidal anti-inflammatory drug [NSAID] that directly targets COX-2, an enzyme responsible for inflammation and pain), minimizing osteoarthritis or other chronic inflammatory conditions. On the flip side, use ginger sparingly as it can cause heartburn and gas, make gallstones worse, and it may mess with some medications such as blood thinners.

Turmeric: This bright yellow spice has some solid gold health benefits. It's active ingredient, curcumin, is a potent antioxidant and seems to help fight cancer and even boost chemotherapy's effects and might be beneficial in managing heart disease, diabetes, and Alzheimer's disease. A daily dose can be as effective a pain reliever as ibuprofen. But like all things good for you, too much turmeric might not be a good thing.

It can inhibit blood clotting in large doses, may intensify gallbladder issues, and has been known to turn the mouth and teeth bright yellow when heavily ingested. Also, the antioxidants don't travel well, so you need to find fresh root to make the most of its many health pluses.

Fresh Herbs: Research has shown that the traditional Mediterranean diet reduces the risk of heart disease, but the herbs used in cooking the foods have their own unique health benefits (sorry, no wine included). Rosemary helps soothe digestion problems such as heartburn, gas, and gallbladder complaints. Thyme has antimicrobial properties that can squash food poisoning, staph, and E. coli, and is also a good digestion aid. Oregano also has antibacterial and antifungal properties that make it effective against some forms of food-borne illnesses, yeast-based infections like vaginitis and oral thrush, and even some antibiotic-resistant infections. Basil has anti-cancer, anti-viral, and anti-microbial abilities, as well as high amounts of a compound that selectively binds the cannabinoid receptor CB2, blocking inflammation pathways without mood-altering effects. Sage has been shown to help with memory and mood and its estrogen-like effects might help curb hot flashes and other symptoms in menopausal women. Fresh is best with all of these herbs. To keep them fresh for about a week, trim the stems and stick in a glass of water loosely covered with a plastic bag.

Salt: It has no claim to healthy fame and you don't want to overdo it, or do it at all if you're on a low-sodium diet, but a pinch of salt can bring out the complex flavors in your green smoothie (a handful of salty veggies like celery or chard will have a similar effect).

Vanilla Extract: Another no-real-health-benefit additive. However, it's the secret ingredient that made nearly everything mom baked taste better. A couple of drops will do the same for your green smoothie. Make sure you use real extract and check the ingredients as even 100 percent pure can have added corn syrup (see page 92 to make your own).

Sweet Indulgences

There are many alternatives other than refined sugar if you want to add a little more sweetness to your green smoothie. But sweeten with a light touch. More sugar, whatever its source, means more weight gain. While there's no official RDA for sugar, recent research from the American Heart Association recommends that the daily intake is 5 teaspoons (20 grams) for adult women, 9 teaspoons (36 grams) for adult men, and 3 teaspoons (12 grams) a day for children.

Agave: Pronounced "ah-GAH-vay," this nectar/syrup is made from the same plant that tequila is made from. Unlike the liquor, agave's probiotic properties nourish the gut. A smidgeon higher in calories than sugar, it's also 25 percent sweeter, so you can use less of it.

Coconut Sugar: Its low Glycemic Index and low processing make it a healthier-than-sugar substitute, but its cost means you'll use it a lot more sparingly.

Dark Chocolate: Stick with 70 percent cacao content and above to garner its blood pressure—and heart disease—fighting compounds.

Fruit: Aim for a little of one of the sweeter fruits such as mango.

Honey: Its antifungal and antibacterial properties ward off colds, but its Glycemic Index is higher than agave's.

Maple Syrup: Pure maple syrup is high in antioxidants, zinc—which boosts the immune system—and manganese, necessary for the body's enzyme reactions

Medjool Dates: Medjool dates are a good choice because they come with added fiber and potassium. Make sure they're pitted. Two dates should be enough.

Molasses: A by-product of sugarcane processing, it has a surprising nutritional value (especially if its blackstrap) and can bundle about 20 percent of your RDA for iron and as much calcium as half a glass of milk. However, its strong taste means it can only be used sparingly.

Raw or Turbinado Sugar: Minimally processed cane sugar; unlike white or brown sugar, it will have a high molasses content.

Stevia: Less is more with this plant-derived sweetener. While it's up to 300 times sweeter than sugar, it's zero calories and doesn't cause a spike in blood glucose levels, sparing you the crash that often follows a spoonful of sugar. Experiment with different brands, as some have a bitter or liquorice aftertaste.

Pour the Foundation

The best liquid you can add to your green smoothie is water. But these fluids will also add an ultrasmooth consistency to your drink:

- For a thicker shake-like vibe, blend in crushed ice.

- A spoonful of sour cream will give your green smoothie a creamier texture.

- A teaspoon of extra-virgin olive oil, coconut oil, fish oil, cod oil, or evening primrose oil will keep things squeaky smooth.

- Nut milk (page 91) like almond or coconut is healthier than cow's milk because its fats are plant-based.

- Coconut water is an even better choice than nut milk as it's lower in calories.

- Add a fermented flavor with a kombucha brew (page 89).

- The natural sweetness of fruit juices like orange, blueberry, apple, cranberry, and pomegranate means you definitely won't want to add any other sugar.

Add-In Cheat Sheet

When you want to counteract that midnight fried feast: Throw in ¼ of an avocado. This green fruit's creamy texture and satisfying flavor can also lower your risk of heart disease by reducing bad cholesterol (LDL) and increasing good cholesterol (HDL).

When your (insert annoying relative) is visiting: Throw in a tomato. It helps to keep blood pressure in check and reduce the number of free radicals in the body.

When it's a high smog alert day: Throw in broccoli sprouts. Broccoli is great for your health, but the prepubescent sprout version (i.e., broccoli plants that are only about five days old) contains high levels of sulforaphane, a compound that increases the production of antioxidant enzymes in airways, which help to prevent inflammation and, potentially, asthma.

When you're feeling run down: Throw in some broccoli spears. This vegetable deserves its crown—it's an all-around superfood that is low in calories (about 30 calories per cup) and high in health-promoting antioxidants, beta-carotene, vitamin C, and folate that can combat the risk of stomach, lung, and rectal cancers and heart disease, ward off cataracts, boost immunity to colds and flus, and reduce the risk of birth defects.

When you have a hot date: Throw in some carrots. These orange wonders are loaded with eye, skin, and hair-enriching nutrients. But don't eat too many in an attempt to smooth out the crow's feet—overdosing on carrots can cause the skin to turn a little orange, which isn't a good look.

When you need an instant detox: Throw in a radish. These root vegetables may help to purify the blood and raise oxygen levels and act as a natural diuretic, helping with kidney and liver function and urinary disorders.

When you're in the mood for a banana split: Throw in ¼ of an avocado or ½ of a banana to make your green smoothie Häagen Dazs creamy.

When you feel a cold coming on: Throw in some chile peppers. They are a quick-acting immunity booster. Plus the spicy heat will make you forget any other ailments!

When you think you might have a UTI: Throw in some cranberry or pomegranate juice, which has been found to actually cure this social calendar–dampening infection.

When you have a yeast infection: Throw in some yogurt, which has been shown to balance the bacteria in our digestive tract.

When you have a sore muscle that just won't stop aching: Throw in some olive oil. One study found that it's as effective as ibuprofun at reducing inflammation.

When you can't remember your boss' kids' names: Throw in some turmeric. Studies show that it inhibits the growth of plaques associated with Alzheimer's.

When you just can't poop: Throw in some whole grains. They're high in fiber, which calms inflamed tissues while keeping the colon healthy.

When you can't find your glasses: Throw in a yellow squash. Carrots may help Bugs Bunny spot Elmer Fudd, but yellow squash contains three specific plant pigments that help to put life into perspective: lutein and xanthine scavenge the free radicals (unstable molecules born from pollution and stress, which can damage cells) that cause eye diseases such as cataracts, while beta-carotene (which converts to vitamin A, stored in the eye) sheds light on night vision.

When you finish the kids' Halloween candy…before November 1: Throw in a sweet potato. Unlike white potatoes, which can actually cause blood sugar to boom, the orange tubers are called the "anti-diabetic" veg because they have a stabilizing effect on sugar levels and even lessen insulin resistance. They're also a good source of fiber and iron, so not only do they give you energy once you come down from your candy high, they can also help regulate the havoc all that processed junk is playing on your digestive system.

When you have a family history of cancer: Throw in a pepper. Red, yellow, orange, or green—a bell pepper a day may keep the Big C away. Studies show that they're rich with nutrients that may lower your risk of developing lung, colon, bladder, and pancreatic cancers.

When you had a heavy sweat session at the gym: Throw in some soybeans. These beans deliver energizing nutrients, particularly B vitamins, copper, and phosphorous, and exercise-friendly carbs, fiber, and protein for muscles.

When you're totally, completely, utterly stressed out: Throw in a stalk of celery—with leaves. Thanks to active phthalides, which relax the muscles of the arteries that regulate blood pressure so the vessels dilate and reduce stress hormones, which can cause blood vessels to constrict, celery is just the prescription for keeping your cool.

When you have a family history of heart disease: Throw in a cuke. Cucumbers contain lariciresinol, pinoresinol, and secoisolariciresinol, three types of lignan chemical compounds that may lower the risk of cardiovascular disease.

When it's the morning after the night after: Instead of the hair of the dog, throw in some hairy artichoke leaves. Antioxidants like cynarin and silymarin make the artichoke an organic detoxifier. It's a natural diuretic, improves gallbladder function, and may even regenerate liver tissue.

When you can't stop burping at the dinner table: Throw in some ginger root. Using ginger for acid reflux has been a popular natural remedy for centuries and has been proven to work for heartburn and other digestive problems.

When you don't have time for a manicure: Throw in some eggs. They're high in sulfur, which helps form strong nails and hair.

When life is getting you down: Throw in some shaved cacao/cocoa. It seems obvious that chocolate will make you feel better, but it actually comes with built-in mood-boosting properties.

When you want to turn your half-empty glass into one that's half full: Throw in some pumpkin seeds. Optimists eat more of the antioxidant carotenoids than people with a negative attitude.

When you want to look buff without going for the burn: Throw in some quinoa. Popeye should have been eating this stuff. Nothing beats pure protein when it comes to building muscle, and quinoa can go nose-to-nose with beef on that count.

When you're wheat-free but long for the nutty taste of grain: Throw in some amaranth. Most seeds are gluten-free, but these kernels are so much like grain that you might think you're drinking a liquefied slice of whole wheat (which tastes better than it sounds).

When you want to stop the PMS: Throw in some sesame seeds, which can alleviate the symptoms connected with this monthly madness.

When you're starting to feel like your sweet old granny: Throw in some pumpkin seeds. Their inflammation-fighting properties can lower the risk of tendinitis, bursitis, arthritis, and gout.

When you're too lazy to go on a diet: Throw in some chia seeds. Unlike flaxseed, chia seeds don't have to be ground (however they break down more easily if they're softened in water before using) and they don't go rancid the way flax does. But they have a similar high fiber content which means they pack a nutritional punch without adding a lot of extra calories to your diet. They will keep you fuller longer and take longer to digest so you'll overeat less and tend to snack less. If you eat chia before a meal, you'll eat less at the next meal.

When you want to make a baby: Throw in some sunflower seeds. Sunflower seeds contain high amounts of zinc, which has been found to be an important mineral for fertility.

When you're in the mood for a protein load but want to miss the acid reflux that can come with carnivorous indulgence: Throw in some tofu. Soy is a light and easily digestible protein but as satisfying as a quarter pounder.

When you can't get rid of the sniffles: Throw in some camu powder. It's high in cold-fighting vitamin C.

When your breath could knock out an army: Throw in some chlorella powder, which will make your mouth fresh for kissing.

When you keep hitting the snooze button: Throw in some protein powder for an instant burst of energy.

When, OMG, you forgot to wash the produce: Throw in some kefir, which has been shown to destroy food-borne infections like E. coli.

Make It, Don't Buy It

It's cheaper to make some of the add-ins mentioned in this chapter yourself, and you guarantee that your from-scratch green smoothie ingredients will contain nothing but what you add so no artificial flavors, preservatives, or coloring will be harmed in the making of your food.

NUTS AND SEEDS PROTEIN POWDER

3 tablespoons raw sesame seeds

3 tablespoons raw flaxseeds

3 tablespoons chlorella or spirulina powder

3 tablespoons chia seeds

3 tablespoons raw peanuts, almonds, or walnuts

Pulverize all the ingredients together into a fine powder in a coffee grinder. This may take up to 5 minutes, depending upon the grinder. Store in an airtight nonmetal container in a cool, dry place.

GRAIN PROTEIN POWDER

   3 tablespoons steel-cut oats

   3 tablespoons brown rice

   3 tablespoons dried green lentils

Pulverize all the ingredients into a fine powder in a coffee grinder. This may take up to 5 minutes, depending upon the grinder. Store in an airtight nonmetal container in a cool, dry place.

VARIATIONS: Unless otherwise stated, grind the main ingredients before adding these. If necessary, grind again until the mix is blended to a fine powder.

   Espresso: I tablespoon whole coffee beans

   Chocolate: I tablespoon unsweetened cacao/cocoa powder, dark chocolate, or cacao/cocoa nibs

   Vanilla: Once the main ingredients are ground, stash a half of a vanilla pod in the container with the powder

   Pumpkin Spice: ¼ teaspoon each of ground ginger and ground cinnamon, and ⅛ teaspoon each of ground nutmeg and ground cloves

   Tropical: I tablespoon coconut flakes (preferably unsweetened)

   Spicy: I tablespoon ground ginger or ⅛ inch fresh ginger root, unpeeled and pulverised

   Salty: I tablespoon crumbled seaweed

NUT BUTTER

   shelled raw nuts of choice (1½ cups of nuts will yield about 1 cup nut butter)

Put the nuts in a food processor or high-powered blender and puree until they become a smooth paste, stopping to scrape the sides of the container as needed. Store in a glass jar in the refrigerator (if the butter hardens, regrind it before using). It will keep for up to 6 months, but you will use it up much more quickly!

VARIATIONS

Chunky Nut Butter: Throw in a handful of nuts once your initial grinding efforts have become a paste. Pulse until it's just how crunchy you like it.

Roasted Nut Butter: Bake the shelled raw nuts on a sheet in a preheated oven at 350°F for 5 to 10 minutes, or cook in a cast-iron pan on medium heat, shaking every few minutes, until fragrant and brown, 3 to 5 minutes. Then grind the nuts.

SEED BUTTER

shelled raw seeds of choice (1 ¼ cups of seeds will yield about 1 cup seed butter)

olive, vegetable, or coconut oil (optional)

salt (optional)

Put the seeds in a food processor or high-powered blender and puree until it becomes a smooth paste, stopping to scrape the sides of the container as needed. Add ½ teaspoon of oil per 1 cup of seeds (if you want to make it creamier, you may need to add a little more or less, depending on the power of your tool) and salt to taste, if desired, and process for 30 seconds more. Store in a glass jar in the refrigerator (if the butter hardens, regrind it before using).

VARIATION

Roasted Seed Butter: Before grinding, toast the seeds in a dry pan over medium heat until fragrant, 1 to 2 minutes.

MILK KEFIR

1 part milk kefir grains (available online or at natural food stores)

8 parts milk (any type)

Stir the kefir grains together with the milk in a clean glass or nonmetallic container. How much milk and kefir grains you want to use is up to you, but a typical ratio is 1 part grains to 8 parts milk. Cover with a cloth (to keep the air flowing through) secured with a rubber band.

Leave the jar at room temperature for about 24 hours. If it's particularly cold in your kitchen, you may want to keep the jar in the warmest spot you can find. Kefir grains prefer warmth.

The mix should be thickened and just starting to separate into curds and whey after 24 hours (you don't want it to completely separate). It may take longer if the room is cold, so leave it out for another 12 to 24 hours if necessary.

Gently stir with a nonmetal spoon to break up the curds and strain through a nonmetallic fine-mesh strainer or cheesecloth. Gently stir the kefir to encourage it to move through the strainer. Store the liquid in an airtight jar in the fridge.

PENNY-PINCHING MOVE: Use the "grains" left in the strainer to start a new batch of kefir, if desired. After a few batches, your kefir grains will start increasing in mass. The kefir will brew in less time when this starts to happen. If the kefir begins to get too thick, you can use more milk for brewing each batch, remove some of the grains to give away, or split your grains to make a second or backup batch of grains.

When you're not making kefir, you can slow-brew the leftover grains in a fresh jar of milk in the fridge. The kefir will ferment very slowly in the fridge, anywhere from a week to several weeks. When you're ready to have kefir, just place at room temperature to continue the brew as usual. If storing in the fridge for a long period of time, strain the grains and "feed" it fresh milk every few weeks. After cold storage, the first brew that you make from the grains at room temperature may take a bit longer as the grains revive. After a few batches at room temperature, the kefir should taste fine.

DAIRY-FREE KEFIR

- 4 to 5 tablespoons sucanat, rapadura, agave nectar, or maple syrup (honey is antibacterial and may slowly kill the grains)
- 1 tablespoon water kefir grains
- 1 quart water (or enough to fill a 2-quart to 1-gallon-size jar while leaving ½ to 1 inch of space at the top)

Shake or stir all of the ingredients in a nonmetallic container until the sugars are completely dissolved. Cover with a cloth secured with a rubber band and allow to brew at room temperature for 24 to 48 hours (or longer). Taste every

12 hours after the first day. If it's too sweet, let it ferment longer. If you forget and it's too sour, you can dilute it with juice or sweetened tea when drinking.

When the kefir is fermented, strain the grains out using a nonmetallic sieve or cheesecloth. Store the finished water kefir in the fridge in a covered jar or in airtight bottles. Storing the water kefir in airtight bottles while the brew is still slightly sweet and allowing to brew in the airtight bottles for a few hours at room temperature will make it fizzy. But don't make the bottles airtight, as the pressure may build and you'll end up with a kefir explosion, which is not a pretty sight.

PENNY-PINCHING MOVE: To resuse the water kefir grains, add 1 to 2 tablespoons of sucanat, rapadura, or molasses, as they need the minerals in those sugars to grow. Cover with water (using twice as much as water as grains) and store at room temperature or in the fridge. If storing at room temperature, change out the liquid for new water and sugar every 2 to 3 days. If storing in the fridge (which will take longer for the grains to brew), change every week.

YOGURT

½ gallon milk (whole or 2% are best, but skim can also be used)

½ cup live yogurt

Heat the milk in a large, heavy saucepan or Dutch oven to just below boiling or, if you have a thermometer, 200°F. Gently stir the milk with a wood spoon as it heats to make sure the bottom doesn't scorch and the milk doesn't boil over. You can also heat it in a microwave-safe container in the microwave for about 3 minutes (you'll need a thermometer to ensure you have reached the right temp; if it's too cool, the yogurt won't set, and if it's too hot, it will turn into curd).

Let the milk cool until it's just hot to the touch, 112°F to 115°F. This goes faster if you set the pan over a bowl of ice and water and gently stir the milk with a wooden spoon.

Pour about 1 cup of the warm milk into a small nonmetallic bowl and whisk it with the yogurt. Once it's smooth, whisk this back into the pan of milk.

Incubate the mixture by warming the oven to about 115°F and then turning off the heat off. Put the lid on the Dutch oven or saucepan and wrap the whole pot in a few layers of towels. These will insulate the pot and keep it warm. Set this bundle in the warmed (but turned off!) oven. It should set for 4 to 6 hours (you can also use a commercial yogurt maker, or some bread makers have a yogurt-making control). It's important not to handle the milk too much so it sets properly—so no early peeks! The texture should be creamy, like a barely-set custard, and the flavor will be tart yet milky. The longer the yogurt sits, the thicker and tangier it will become. Cool the yogurt in the same container in the refrigerator before transferring it into an airtight nonmetallic container. If there's a film of watery whey on top of the yogurt, strain it and save to add to a green smoothie, or stir it back into the yogurt. The yogurt will last about 2 weeks in the refrigerator.

PENNY-PINCHING MOVE: Instead of buying yogurt, save ½ cup of the yogurt you made as the starter yogurt next time.

VARIATION

Greek Yogurt: Prepare the yogurt as instructed. Line a large bowl with several thicknesses of cheesecloth. Add the yogurt, gather the ends of the cloth, and fasten them tightly with a rubber band. Slip the rubber band over the sink faucet or a cupboard knob to hang the bundle and place a bowl underneath. There will be a thin stream of water that comes out immediately, which will slow to a drip. Leave hanging for 8 to 12 hours. Reserve the drained whey to add to add to a green smoothie as a liquid protein base.

RICOTTA

Traditionally, ricotta is made by reheating whey left over from cheese making, but this is a quick cheat's method.

  3 parts whole milk

  1 part distilled white vinegar

  salt, to taste (optional)

Heat the milk in a large, heavy nonreactive pot over medium heat. If you're using salt, stir it in now. Slowly heat the milk until just below boiling, or near scalding temperature (180°F to 185°F), stirring occasionally (steam will start to form above the surface and tiny bubbles will appear). Take the pot off the heat and gently stir in the vinegar. Curds should form immediately. Cover the pot with a clean, dry dish towel and leave the mixture to sit undisturbed.

After 2 or more hours, dampen a piece of cheesecloth and use it to line a nonmetallic colander placed inside a large non-metallic bowl. Gently pour the ricotta into the colander and leave to drain for about 2 hours, depending how creamy or dry you want the cheese to be. Refrigerate in an airtight container for up to 7 days. Reserve the drained whey to add to a green smoothie as a liquid protein base.

COTTAGE CHEESE

1 gallon skim milk

¾ cup white vinegar

1½ teaspoons kosher salt

½ cup half-and-half or heavy cream

Heat the skim milk in a large saucepan over medium heat to 120°F. Remove from the heat and gently add in the vinegar, stirring for a couple of minutes until the curd starts separating from the whey. Cover and let it rest at room temperature for 30 minutes.

Line a colander with cheesecloth and place on a larger bowl. Pour the "cheese" into the colander and let drain for 5 minutes. Gather up the edges of the cloth and rinse under cold water for 3 to 5 minutes or until the curd is completely cooled, gently squeezing the mixture the whole time. Once cooled, squeeze as dry as possible and transfer to a nonmetallic bowl. Add the salt and stir to combine, breaking up the curd into bite-size pieces as you go. If ready to use immediately, stir in the half-and-half or heavy cream. If not, transfer to a sealable container and place in the refrigerator. Add the half and half or heavy cream just prior to using. Reserve the drained whey to add to a green smoothie as a liquid protein base.

AS GOOD AS BUTTERMILK

1 tablespoon white vinegar or lemon juice

1 cup cow's milk (whole, 2%, or heavy cream)

Add the white vinegar or lemon juice to a liquid measuring cup. Add enough milk to bring the liquid up to the 1-cup line. Let stand for 5 minutes and it will thicken to a buttermilk consistency.

KOMBUCHA TEA

Makes about 1 gallon

2 quarts water

½ cup sweetener such as organic sugar or evaporated cane juice (the "tea" needs a non-bacterial sugar to feed, and other types of sugar can make the brew taste sour)

4 bags black tea or 1 tablespoon loose black tea

1 cup unpasteurized, neutral-flavored starter kombucha (available from natural foods store)

1 SCOBY (Symbiotic Colony of Bacteria and Yeast), aka "mother" or "mushroom" (available from natural food stores)

Boil the water and mix with the sugar until it's dissolved. Add the tea and steep for a few hours until the water has cooled. You can speed up the cooling process by placing the pot in bowl of ice water.

Once the tea is cool, remove the tea bags or strain out the loose tea. Stir in the starter kombucha.

Transfer to a large glass jar and add the SCOBY. Cover the mouth of the jar with a few layers of cheesecloth or paper towels secured with a rubber band and leave at room temperature out of direct sunlight for 7 to 10 days, checking occasionally. The SCOBY may float to the top or sink to the bottom. A new, cream-colored layer of SCOBY should start forming on the surface within a few days. It might attach to the old SCOBY or separate. There may also be unappetizing-looking brown stringy bits floating beneath the SCOBY, sediment collecting at the bottom, and/or bubbles collecting around the SCOBY, which are all signs of healthy fermentation.

After 7 days, taste the kombucha daily by pouring a little out of the jar and into a cup. When you're happy with the balance of sweet and tart, it's ready to bottle. First prepare and cool another pot of strong tea for your next batch of kombucha, as outlined above. Then lift the SCOBY out of the kombucha tea and put it aside on a clean plate.

Measure out 1 cup of starter tea and set it aside for the next batch. If you're using flavorings (see Variations below), add now and steep for 2 more days. Strain the fermented (and possibly flavored) kombucha into bottles, leaving about ½ inch of head room in each bottle.

Store the bottled kombucha at room temperature out of direct sunlight for 1 to 3 days for the kombucha to carbonate. Refrigerate to stop fermentation and carbonation and use within 1 month.

In the meantime, start your next batch. Clean the jar being used for kombucha fermentation. Combine the starter tea from your last batch of kombucha with a fresh amount of sugary tea and pour it into the fermentation jar. Slide the SCOBY on top, cover, and ferment for 7 to 10 days.

Even if you're not ready to make more tea, you need to feed and care for your SCOBY (it's like the Chia pet of the 21st century). It can be stored in a fresh batch of the tea base with the starter tea in the fridge. Change out the tea for a fresh batch every 4 to 6 weeks.

VARIATION

Fruit tea instead of black tea: Add 1 cup chopped fruit, 2 cups fruit juice, 1 tablespoons flavored tea (like hibiscus or Earl Grey), 2 tablespoons of honey, 3 tablespoons fresh herbs or spices to the tea before storing.

PENNY-PINCHING MOVE: A purchased SCOBY can be expensive. If you can, beg one off of a kombucha-brewing friend. Or you can make your own using a bottle of organic, raw kombucha drink (available from natural foods stores; it must be raw) and a cup of black tea, sweetened with a tablespoon of sugar. Pour the bottle of kombucha and sweetened tea into a glass jar. Cover it with a towel so it can breathe but be protected from insects and other contaminants. Let it sit in a dark, warm spot for about 2 to 3 weeks (depending on the room temperature). A SCOBY will start to form on top of the liquid. It will appear first as a thin film, then slowly fill in and thicken up. Once it's about ¼ inch thick, it's ready to use.

Caring for Your SCOBY

A SCOBY will last a very long time, but it's not indestructible. To prolong its life, peel off the bottom (oldest) layer every few batches. This can be discarded, composted, or used to start a new batch of kombucha. If it becomes black, it has passed its lifespan. If it has green or black mold, it has become infected. Either way, throw it away and begin again.

NUT OR SEED MILK

   1 part nuts or seeds (almonds work really well, but cashews, Brazil
      nuts, hazelnuts, macadamias, pecans, pistachios, and walnuts or even
      seeds like hemp, sunflower, flax, chia, pumpkin, sesame, and pine
      "nuts" may also be used)

   2 parts water

Soak the nuts or seeds overnight. In addition to making them tender, soaking de-activates the compounds that keep the nuts or seeds dormant, and activates the enzymes that make them sprout and the nutrients more easily digested.

Drain the water and rinse the nuts or seeds well before using and then mix with a new batch of water, this time using a ratio of 3:1 or 3 cups of water for each cup of presoaked nuts or seeds. If you prefer a thicker, richer milk, decrease the amount of water to your liking. Process or blend until the nuts or seeds are very finely ground and the water has turned a light milky color. Strain through a layer of cheesecloth.

PENNY-PINCHING MOVE: Don't strain the milk. That pulp isn't compost; it will add thickness to your smoothie, and the high-fiber content means you can save on fiber supplements.

COCONUT MILK

¼ cup dried, shredded, or desiccated coconut

1 cup water

Combine the coconut and water well in a blender or food processor. Pour into a glass bowl lined with a nut milk bag or cheese cloth, and strain to remove the pulp.

PENNY-PINCHING MOVE: Skip the straining step—the pulp will thicken your green smoothie without having to buy extra ingredients and the extra fiber will take the place of any supplements you might use.

VANILLA EXTRACT

2 vanilla bean pods

1 pint (2 cups) vodka

Add the pods to the vodka and let sit in a dark cool place for a few months. The vodka should turn slightly darker. Remove the pods before using as you would any vanilla extract.

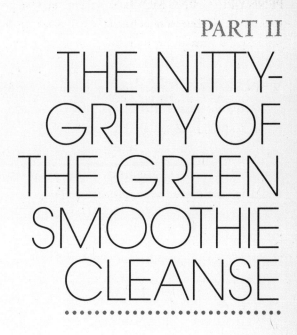

PART II

THE NITTY-GRITTY OF THE GREEN SMOOTHIE CLEANSE

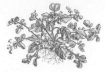

CHAPTER SEVEN

Getting Clean

A green smoothie cleanse is a regimen of eating—or rather, drinking—that eliminates alcohol and caffeine, limits meat and dairy such as butter and hard cheeses, and focuses instead on fresh whole foods such as vegetables and fruits as well as nuts, beans, whole grains, and water.

·That's it.

The smoothies are simple and quick to make. They don't require purchasing special powders, supplements, or anything other than a few pounds of fruit, vegetables, and protein such as nuts or yogurt. This is major when you consider that smoothie bars alone have become a $2 billion industry and there seem to be as many places to stock up on cleansing kits as there are stores to buy skinny jeans. But you don't have to invest in a salary check's worth of premade drinks or smoothie mixes or even a special blender to go on a green smoothie cleanse or even get your Greenster creds.

However, this is an extremely healthy drink; not a miracle cure.

This means that a green smoothie cleanse probably won't remove toxins from your body. But that's because there isn't really anything to detox. This holds true even if you have overloaded your body with fat, alcohol, and microwave meals and slept on a mattress soaked in flame-retardant and stain-resistant chemicals situated in a public restroom every day for the past year. The fact is that our bodies have a 100 percent proven way to detox themselves. To put it in technical terms, we poop, pee, breathe, and sweat. What a green smoothie cleanse can do is keep the kidneys, liver, and intestines tuned-up in the same way that an oil change keeps your car engine running smoothly. Too much alcohol, fatty foods, and sodium and too little water can keep these detox organs operating at the best.

Another thing a green smoothie cleanse won't do is boost your immune system, dry up your sniffles, or treat any other disease. The only way to directly affect your immune system is to expose it to an infection; what's called the adaptive part of your system will then develop protective killer cells in response. However, because a green smoothie cleanse keeps your diet healthy in a deluge of nutrient-rich vegetables and fruit, the spillover effect is that your body will have all the essential vitamins and minerals it needs to keep everything working well.

The other big question is if you'll you lose weight on the green smoothie cleanse. Probably, but that's because you'll be cutting out a lot of foods from your diet and lowering your caloric intake. You will also probably gain some back after you go off the cleanse. That is to be expected and is actually healthy, since regularly depriving your body of energy can have the boomerang effect of lowering your metabolism permanently.

Losing weight isn't about not eating food. (If you want to drop 20 pounds instantly, cut off a leg.) Your body wants, expects, needs, and deserves food. Successfully changing your size is about eating more quality food. The green smoothie cleanse—unlike most other cleanses—includes eating foods with two ingredients mandatory for doing this: protein, which helps maintain muscle mass and energy levels during weight loss, and dietary fiber, which acts as a healthy stomach filler. This also means that the cleanse can safely be followed long-term.

The idea is to give yourself a mental jump start to eating better. The fact is, almost everyone's diet could stand some improvement. Eating healthfully is a conscious, ongoing commitment. A green smoothie cleanse will make you not just think about food, but think differently about the food you put into your body and, as a result, hopefully permanently improve your eating habits and prepare your body for a more active and healthier life. Think of it as a clean living reboot, a way to a caffeine-free, veggie- and fruit-filled, de-stressed, totally buff new you.

Go Cleanse Yourself

You can have a green smoothie anytime. But should you actually go on a green smoothie cleansing program? Answer yes to more than two of the following questions and the answer is yes, you probably need to cleanse up your life:

- Do you seem to always have a zit flare-up?
- Do you fall asleep while watching TV at night?
- Do you have a tough time getting up in the morning?
- Do you have a case of sniffles you just can't shake?
- Do you have difficulty pooping regularly (once a day or every other day)?
- Has it been more than a day since you last ate a vegetable (ketchup does not count) or fruit?
- Does it seem like it would be easier to repeat high school algebra than lose a few pounds?
- Do you look like you have raccoon eyes?
- Do you often feel as bloated as the blow-up Shrek in the Macy's Thanksgiving parade?
- Does your brain sometimes feel so foggy that you forget deadlines or your dog's birthday?
- Does your breath make even your dentist reel?

- Does it feel like your brain is in constant Must Have Sugar mode?
- Does your body regularly glisten more than the models in a Calvin Klein underwear ad—even when you aren't working out and the temperature is below sauna level?
- Do you often experience headaches that feel like a herd of elephants is using your brain for *Stomp* practice?
- Are antacid pills a part of your daily diet?

If you qualify for a cleanse, don't dust off your blender just yet. If you can't answer "yes" to *all* of the following, wait until you can. You will be a happier and definitely more successful green smoothie cleanser as a result:

- You'll have easy access to a bathroom for the duration of the cleanse.
- There are no houseguests or family events in your immediate future.
- Your work schedule is clear and you don't have any big projects due soon.
- If you're a woman, you're not due to get your period just before or during the cleanse and you're not pregnant or nursing (while green smoothies are a deliciously nutritious supplement to a pregnancy diet, a cleanse simply cannot give you the boatload of calories you need to help your baby grow).
- You don't have a getaway booked. Really? Carrying around jars of green liquid (presuming you can even make the drink) is how you want to spend your summer vacation?
- You have not already cleansed four times this year. Yes, the green smoothie cleanse is one of the healthiest cleanses out there, but you can have too much of even a good thing.

If you're good to go and you're hungry to know what to expect when you're cleansing, here's the really good, the so-so, and the just plain ugly of a typical green smoothie cleanse experience.

The Really Good

You realize how much your life is dominated by what you put in your mouth. Food is so much a part of our daily rites and rituals. In fact, our lives often revolve around our next meal. Whether we're eating in or out, those three meals a day are a focal point of our day. It's amazing how many hours a day we spend thinking about, shopping for, putting away, preparing, cooking, and cleaning up after the food in our lives. Whether we're welcoming a new family member, witnessing the creation of a new bond, or saying good-bye to someone special, food is not only what sustains us—it is the thing that brings us together, nurturing us and bringing us comfort and celebrating our joy.

Switching to green smoothies for a set period helps you recognize your own personal eating emotional subtext. For three or more days, you won't have any food dilemmas other than how much green smoothie you want to put into your cup or water bottle. You may begin to realize how important food is to you on a personal level. You might discover that you're using food as a stress reducer or a quick energy fix. Or you might find that your need to keep your bathing suit figure is harder work than you had anticipated. The stress attached to dieting can be just as detrimental as the stress of being overweight. In both cases, food becomes an object to be controlled and manipulated. But on a green smoothie cleanse, it's simply fuel. So with every sip of green smoothie, you're taking control of your life.

A green smoothie cleanse can clear the mind and refresh and regenerate your spiritual willpower by pushing you out of the comfort zone of your daily patterns. Many religions limit the intake of food at various times throughout the year to create a stronger connection with the sacred self.

The green smoothie cleanse isn't a diet. It's a plan to change eating habits long-term. The reason this is in the good category is because most diets fail miserably, usually for the simple reason that they tend to be extremely limiting, not just in terms of how many (or perhaps that should be "few") calories you're allowed to consume, but also with regards to which food groups you can choose from. As a result, they make your body fatter (and extremely tired and cranky) in the long run because your digestive system goes into panic mode and begins storing excess calories. On the other hand, the only foods the green smoothie cleanse restricts are the processed kind. Beyond that, you're actually encouraged to eat more vegetables and more fruit and a little protein— pretty much the USDA's recommended foundation of a healthy diet.

You will glow. One consistently reported anecdotal side effect of the green smoothie cleanse is healthy, radiant skin—no surgery required. This could be the result of not eating processed foods and digesting more fruits and vegetables rich in vitamin C (critical for strong, healthy skin because of its role in the body's manufacture of collagen, a protein that keeps the skin supple and tight; even a slight deficiency can compromise the production of collagen), vitamin E (thought to help in the fight against free radicals), and vitamin A, thiamine, and zinc (all are important for normal cellular function in the skin), and selenium (helps protect the skin from free radicals).

When you're done, you'll feel an amazing sense of accomplishment (plus the joy of thumbing your nose at the "thoughtful" colleague who kept on leaving bags of chips on your desk).

You'll have more mental downtime because you'll free up all those minutes wasted calculating if you're eating enough vegetables. You are.

Quadruple that "me" time if you're putting your family on the cleanse as well. (Your kids can drink the smoothies and it's a simple way to up their vegetable intake, but they should not go on a cleanse without medical supervision, as they need a lot more calories than adults to healthily get through their day.) For once, you know your nearest and dearest are eating all of their required greens.

You'll have more time because green smoothies are essentially one-bowl meals, so they're easy to make and clean up after. No cooking or washing pots!

You'll have more money because you won't have to buy vitamin supplements anymore.

You won't have the morning-after guilt-a-thon that follows a late night snack-a-thon anymore—because you won't have those cravings. Processed foods come packaged with a large amount of fat, sugar, and salt that affect your brain's chemistry, making you want more and more, even when you aren't hungry. Just thinking about or seeing an image of a food high in fat, sugar, or salt can cause you to want to devour it. This addiction response is called "conditioned hyper-eating." In fact, sugar and fat release the same chemicals in your brain involved in drug, alcohol, and gambling addictions. But the green smoothie cleanse helps you kick the habit.

It doesn't matter if you have a presidential dislike for a certain vegetable like Brussels sprouts (Reagan), broccoli (George H. Bush), or beets (Obama). The 60:40 fruit-to-vegetable ratio of a green smoothie means that you will barely even taste the stuff you don't care for.

That little stomach pooch you tell yourself you could lose in a millisecond if you really got serious about it, yet never do? It will be totally gone in a few days.

A green smoothie cleanse effectively gives you a dietary clean slate, which, if you pay attention to how your body reacts to your smoothie ingredients and if you have been varying what goes in your blends, will make it easy to figure out which foods work well for your body.

Even if you rival Calvin of *Calvin and Hobbes* in your dislike of vegetables, you'll have a list of favorite greens within days of going on the green smoothie cleanse.

After a few days, you'll experience a mental high that will annoy those near and dear who aren't also on a green smoothie cleanse, and you'll have enough get-up-and-go to give the Energizer Bunny a run for its money.

It's the perfect excuse: Initially, a cleanse can make your brain foggy. Before this happens, memorize this all-purpose, get-out-of-jail-free phrase: "I'm sorry (insert appropriate situation: I forgot your birthday/forgot our anniversary/was late for our date/made a mistake/can't remember your name/didn't pick up milk/forgot to get gas, etc...), I'm on a cleanse."

The So-So

Remember that little stomach pooch you tell yourself you could lose in a millisecond if you really got serious about it, yet never do? It may come back slightly once the cleanse is over. But at least now you know that it doesn't have to be a permanent part of your landscape.

Even with the fruit, there's no getting around that you're living on a diet of liquidized salad. By somewhere around your eighth green smoothie, you will be SO. TIRED. OF. LIQUID. MEALS. But by your twelfth or so, you'll no longer care.

If you're a daily caffeine drinker, you'll miss your morning jolt in the early days, and the sight of your coffee maker or tea kettle might make you cry.

There is always going to be a family member or colleague who thinks it's funny to text you pictures of hamburgers and chocolate cake or take bets that you won't last more than however many hours.

It's going to take time to figure out what works for you. So if you really can't stand the taste of today's smoothie du jour, don't toss in your salad spinner and call it a day. Play with your flavors and ratios. Add some sweeteners or try some nuts or yogurt to change the consistency. It may take a few tries to find a recipe proportion that works for you. Once you become accustomed to the taste and texture, you can adjust to a more hardcore greens-to-fruit ratio.

Even though you can and should vary the ingredients, it gets boring drinking your meals after while. But the upside is that your hunger will help you to ID your eating pitfalls quickly, like if you're overdoing it on portion size and reaching for food simply out of boredom, or because someone within a five mile radius is eating.

Initially your stomach will growl. Just hope it isn't during an important meeting.

Meeting friends for drinks will be tough.

There will be times when you'll feel deprived, hungry, and cranky (in cleanse parlance, "hangry"). Or keeping to the cleanse will be inconvenient. You might be tempted to cheat and you might follow through. But don't feel guilty. Just get back on your smoothie schedule. This isn't a diet; it's a path to healthier eating. So even if you do slip up, chances are once the cleanse is over you won't start inhaling every cookie and chip within reach.

You will really appreciate even the subtlest of whole food flavors. The cameo that cinnamon, for instance, makes in a day filled with spinach and cabbage can feel like a Pop Rocks explosion in your mouth.

The Just Plain Ugly

You may not feel any different. The effects of a green smoothie cleanse aren't like one of those magic potions from a fairy tale. Even if you don't notice the effects, eating a purer diet is having a positive effect on your body. It may take a while, but eventually you'll realize that you have more energy and get-up-and-go.

You do feel different: You feel awful. You might feel so sick to your stomach after swigging your green smoothie that the thought of drinking another in a few hours makes you want to whimper or gag. Chances are that these feelings will pass in a few days. But if you really can't stomach it, then forget the actual cleanse for now. Instead, reduce the amount of smoothies you're preparing to one a day and gradually work yourself up to more. At the same time, try to "cleanse" the other food you're eating—leave out meat and anything processed if possible (even for just a matter of a few weeks). Think of it as cleanse light—all the benefits of a regular green smoothie cleanse, but with slower results. Not to worry. After all, this isn't about a quick fix. It's about developing a long-term habit of healthy eating, and that isn't going to happen over-night. Later on, once you have become more used to the drink regimen, you can try a full-fledged cleanse again.

You might feel cranky and lethargic at first. Or have a mild head-ache, excess mucous, an acne emergency, or stomach aches. Honest, this is all good stuff. These symptoms are what comes form switching to a mostly plant, all-liquid diet and usually shifts after a few days (see The Really Good, page 98).

Gag! Choking is most likely in your future. A green smoothie is a taste most people need to ease into. Some people find the taste metallic or the texture or aroma swampy. There are a few things you can do to make the smoothie more palatable: Pour it back in the blender and purify, add some fruit juice to make it sweeter and thinner, or slip a banana in to make the texture creamier.

You may feel like you're starving. Try adding some protein to help fill you up. On the downside, our bodies are very adaptive and used to expecting whatever amount we feed them—even when it's, as is often the case, unhealthily too much. On the upside, those adaptive powers mean that your body will also quickly get used to a green smoothie diet.

Day Three. If you're in it for the long-term, then be prepared: The third day of the green smoothie cleanse is the worst. This is the day where you feel really awful and break down and start looking for the powdered donuts. Stay focused and you will feel fantastic. To get through the next 24 hours, choose green smoothie recipes with a flavor that you really like (for example, if you have a sweet tooth, go for ones that are packed with fruits).

You'll have bad breath. Really bad breath. Think a cat on a bad day.

You may feel slightly nauseous and headachy for the first day or two. This comes from switching to a liquid diet. Suck it up, buttercup. You'll feel better in a few days. Whatever you do, don't take any type of painkiller as it will feel awful on your stomach.

You won't be able to get anything done because you'll have to go to the bathroom a lot. To both poop and pee. And expect your bowels to be on the loose side.

Expect bloating and gas. You're packing in a lot more produce than you usually would in a normal meal, which can initially play like a Riverdance on your intestines. It will take a few days for your digestive tract to re-regulate and settle down.

Green stools. Green in, green out.

CHAPTER EIGHT

Simple Strategies for a Successful Cleanse

By now you have hopefully figured out that green smoothies are a great addition to a healthy eating regime. Getting on that healthy diet in the first place is where the green smoothie cleanse comes in. The key to a green smoothie cleanse is basically: Eat more veggies and fruit and eliminate the processed junk.

This sounds simple enough, but in the context of real life and its demands, it can be anything but. After all, this isn't just about getting clean for a specific time frame; it's about using the cleanse to permanently change your eating ways. So getting weighed down with a long list of do's and don'ts isn't going to be helpful in the long-term. Instead, here are some simple strategies that you can easily fit into your daily routine to take the challenge out of cleansing.

Strategy 1:
Put Your Mind Where Your Mouth Is

We often resolve to change our eating habits reactively—after a binge of late night snacking or a season of festive fare—as opposed to proactively. The result? According to studies, most of us slip back into our poor diets within a couple of weeks.

To have a successful green smoothie cleanse, you need to be pro-active and get your head in the game before you shop for kale. Ask yourself why you want to go on a cleanse. It may be to fit into a specific outfit, clean out your system, kick your takeaway dinner habit—it doesn't matter. Being honest about your reasons helps you get (and stay) motivated.

Next, select your start date. Make sure you have enough time to buy the groceries you'll need and that there are no big events like your best friend's wedding or a vacation in Italy that can derail you.

Last, repeat three times: Food is fuel. In other words, food isn't a comfy blanket or a reward or a boredom reliever. If you tend to reach for a chocolate bar after you have a fight with your partner or like to celebrate the events in your life with a meal or even if you tend to chip dip when zoning out during late night TV, it's going to be difficult to make it through your green smoothie cleanse. To take the mood out of your meals, write down a list of potential distractions from fridge forays: calling a friend, cleaning the house, blasting bad '80s tunes on your iPod. When you're tempted to turn to food as an emotional response, put something on your list in play.

Strategy 2: Don't Make a Shopping List

Most cleanses advise you to make a specific list and stick to it. That can make you feel boxed in and unsatisfied. After a while, when you can't stand eating the same foods over and over again, you polish off a pint of ice cream or half a pizza and feel terrible. You really only need to think about the categories of food that you need on the green smoothie diet, like vegetables, fruit, and protein. If kale, bananas, and yogurt are on your shopping list, that's what you'll buy. But if you just write "greens," you'll get what catches your eye—perhaps baby spinach or bok choy.

Strategy 3: Get Zen

Around the second to third day of your cleanse, you'll experience a plateau for a couple of days. You might stop dropping pounds or you may feel a bit draggy or even sick. If you know this is coming, you will (hopefully) not panic.

Strategy 4: Remember to Add

It's a good thing that green smoothies help clarify the mind, because you'll need to keep track of numbers at the beginning. (As you become an old cleanse hand, you'll be able to lose the measuring cups and throw together delicious smoothies by eye.)

You may think you want to jump in with blender revving and a refrigerator full of ingredients that could feed a minivan full of vegetarians for a week. Start with one 16-ounce glass. That may not sound like very much, but you'll feel challenged. Changing your eating habits is all about making small adjustments that are doable; otherwise, while you might be able to stick with a cleanse for a few days or even a few weeks, chances are you'll soon revert back to your pre-cleanse eating ways.

Also, keep to that ratio of 60 percent fruit to 40 percent leafy greens. And begin with the milder-tasting greens. This flavor combo will make it easier to stick with the plan. As your cleanse continues and you drink more green smoothies each day, you'll be able to add more greens and less fruit.

Once you're ready to commit to a cleanse, you'll have a few more calculations. First, aim for at least 1,000 calories initially. While you can definitely have more, less will throw off your metabolism (translation: your body will sound the starvation red alert and begin to hoard every calorie consumed).

Make sure you add protein. While it isn't necessarily a staple if you're making green smoothies an additional part of your daily diet, that extra energy boost is going to be a must when you're on a cleanse. In addition, if you're not feeding your body enough protein, it will have a backlash effect on all the good things a cleanse can do: A diet low in protein can cause unhealthy skin, irritability, lethargy, apathy, muscle wasting, and many bad hair days.

Always count on a little extra zest to get you through the day when you're cleansing. While greens and fruit form the bulk and flavor of your green smoothie, the seasonings that you throw in can determine how easy it will be for you to stick with the plan. Spices can pack a savory punch that will help you feel satisfied, while protein will make you feel fuller for longer.

Last, add up your days. Your cleanse will make you feel so good that you may want to rush and repeat the experience. Resist the urge. The rule of thumb is one day a week for the one day cleanse, one a month for the three-day cleanse, and for anything lasting five days or longer, four times a year, with a three-month waiting period in between each cleanse.

Strategy 5: Don't Chug

Slowly sipping and chewing your smoothies will make you more mindful of what you're putting in your body. It's a good way to become more aware of the tastes and textures of your drink, and it gives your brain time to register that you're full and keep your blood sugars on even keel all day. Don't rush your smoothie time or detract from it by multitasking while you drink. Don't watch TV, read (even this book!), or talk on the phone when drinking. You want to focus on your smoothie. Take small sips and savor the experience. Try to make each "meal" last for at least an hour.

Strategy 6: Keep Your Head in the Game

Don't think of your green smoothie cleanse as something you have to get through or your short-term backup for counteracting your usual unhealthy eating ways. Instead, focus on how great you feel (which you will feel, after a few days), how much better you're sleeping, and how much more energy you seem to have. A positive attitude is an essential ingredient for rebuilding your diet.

Strategy 7: Have an After Plan

Your cleanse is a starting point, not a finish line. So it helps to decide before you begin what you're going to do once it's over and you start to reintroduce foods that you avoided on the cleanse. Don't do it all at once. Instead, add foods into your meals one at a time, every two days. Not only will your body thank you, but a slow and steady approach gives you a chance to monitor your reaction to different kinds of food and possibly identify things you might be sensitive to or that cause you digestive problems.

Strategy 8:
Make a Good Match

Although you'll lose some pounds on a green smoothie cleanse, it isn't inherently a weight-loss diet, but rather a lifestyle choice. So choose the cleanse that best fits your daily needs. Bottom line: The best cleanse is one you can follow.

*Disclaimer: Consult a medical professional before starting a green smoothie cleanse, as some health conditions may be aggravated by the regimen.

CHAPTER NINE

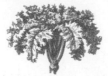

Choose Your Program

A green smoothie cleanse can safely last from a day to a full two weeks (some people follow it for longer, but it isn't advisable or actually even necessary). The time commitment is actually going to be longer than the fast itself since there's prep work before to ease you into the cleanse and the transition period after the cleanse to ease you back into regular eating. The length of both of these time frames is going to depend on the length of your actual cleanse (see the next chapter for more on the whys, wherefores, and hows of cleanse preparation).

Regardless of the duration, however, all green smoothie cleanses are going to have the same positive long-term effect in that they help you to eat greener. Still, there's no such thing as a one-size-fits-all green smoothie cleanse. To help you figure out which cleanse will fit your life right now, answer the following:

1. Is this your first cleanse?   Yes / No

2. Will this be the first time you have   Yes / No
   ever done a green smoothie cleanse?

3. Do you avoid veggies like they are a   Yes / Mostly / No
   coming plague?

4. Do you think fruit is a bad   Yes / Somewhat / No
   substitute for candy?

5. Do you say "Cheers!" with a glass of wine or beer or a cocktail a few times a week?　Yes / Often / No

6. Do you regularly smoke cigarettes?　Yes / No

7. Are you a red-blooded carnivore?　Yes / No

8. Are your meals often on the pale side (white sugar, flour, bread, pasta, cookies, crackers, rice)?　Yes / Mostly / No

9. Is the only water you consume from coffee, tea, and sodas?　Yes / Often / No

10. Are most of your weekly meals made somewhere other than a home kitchen?　Yes / Often / No

11. Is the only sweat you regularly break when running out the door at the end of work?　Yes / Often / No

12. Do you think pizza contains most of the food groups?　Yes / No

13. Do you need a little sugar pick-me-up to get you through the midafternoon slump?　Yes / Often / No

14. Does life have no meaning until you have your morning jolt of caffeine?　Yes / No

Choose Your Cleanse

If you answered "Yes," "Often," "Mostly," or "Somewhat" to nine or more questions, start slow with the One-Day Reboot Cleanse for the first few cleanses to get on a healthier track. A commitment of 24 hours (actually more like 10 hours since you'll need—really need—to sleep) is easy to accomplish and will get you acquainted you with the cleansing process. Instead of focusing on what you aren't eating at this moment that you usually would, use this first experience to find out what *your* body's particular reactions are. Every body is unique, and the more you learn about yours, the easier cleansing becomes.

If you answered anything other than "No" to six to eight questions, still start with a One-Day Reboot Cleanse initially, but go ahead and take your cleansing to the next level the next time with a Three-Day Blast.

If you answered "Yes," "Often," "Mostly," or "Somewhat" to two to five questions, you can kick off with a Five-Day Fine-Tune as long as you checked "No" for the first two questions. Otherwise, stick with a One-Day Reboot Cleanse or Three-Day Blast for the first time. Either way, stay flexible. Keep your five-day goal in mind, but if you end up having a difficult time, it's better to back off into the Three-Day Blast than give up altogether.

If you answered "No" to everything, the smoothie world is your tempeh oyster. You're a Greenster in the making. While it seems like your brass cleanse ring would be a Two-Week Full-Body one, you are better off wading into the world of cleansing and using the Five-Day Fine-Tune as your starting point if you have had at least three previous cleansing experiences; go with a Three-Day Blast if you have only cleansed a couple of times.

Once you have a few cleanses under your belt, the program you choose is going to depend on your lifestyle and immediate goals. What plan can you honestly live with? Keep in mind that the plan you choose today might be different from what you would opt for the next time you want to cleanse. So if the timeframe you decide on isn't for you, don't throw in the towel—or the vegetable peeler. Wait a couple of weeks and then try a different plan.

Note that while these are the most common lengths for cleansing, any amount of time can be chosen, depending on your needs.

Be a Goal-Getter

Once you know what you want out of your cleanse, it's a short chop, blend, and sip to knowing which cleanse is best for you. If:

You want some R&R&R: You have been working hard and playing harder. To recharge, rejuvenate, and renew, make time for a Two-Week Full-Body Cleanse.

Your body type leans toward big hips and wide shoulders: This body type can tend toward sluggishness. A One-Day Reboot Cleanse will get you back on track.

Your body is stocky but strong: You need to regroup with a Three-Day Blast to feel in the best of shape.

You find it difficult to put on weight: When you can eat anything you want, you usually do. While all the cleanses will whittle away at your junk food habit, a Five-Day Fine-Tune is the most likely to really crack it long-term, if not forever.

You want to look better naked—fast: A Three-Day Blast will help you drop some water weight without feeling deprived or hungry.

You need a healthy eating tune-up: The liquefied diet of any of the cleanses is enough to make you crave a salad or a nice bowl of chewy grains, but the inner work of a Five-Day Fine-Tune puts you in a healthier frame of mind as well.

You want to remake your diet and body into a new, improved you: Commit to a Two-Week Full-Body Cleanse for long-lasting changes.

You're preparing for or recovering from seasonal eating: Vacations, holidays, and big events like weddings can wreak havoc on our diets. A Three-Day Blast will work quick wonders, but you'll need to put in effort to make those permanent. For a longer-lasting new, improved you, the Five-Day Fine-Tune is enough time for you to give yourself a mini mind-body makeover.

You're trying to figure out your bad food triggers: A Two-Week Full-Body Cleanse will give you a clean slate for slowly reintroducing foods and deciphering which might be causing you problems.

You're not sure you can do this: One day a week for a few weeks is all you need for some powerful cleansing confidence.

You're a loner: Since you won't be exposed to social pressures, you can probably easily go the distance with a Two-Week Cleanse.

The Cleanse Defined

Here is a rough outline of what you're committing to when you decide to do a green smoothie cleanse. Some of the exact details will change, depending on which cleanse you do:

- A minimum of the recommended green smoothies per day for the length of the cleanse. You can have more if you need them, but you need to have at least the total number set for that cleanse.
- No alcohol.
- No nicotine.
- Only prescribed drugs.
- Some dairy, depending on the cleanse.
- No meat of any kind.
- No processed foods whatsoever.
- No sweeteners other than a small amount of agave, stevia, or honey (depending on the cleanse).
- No legumes or grains, depending on the cleanse.
- Drink a lot of water.
- Drink hot lemon water and/or ginger tea.
- Infuse water with tasty things like lemon, cucumbers, and/or mint (depending on the cleanse).

You like to travel in a herd: Choose a One-Day Reboot Cleanse or a Three-Day Blast. The longer you cleanse, the more difficult it is to do it without having a posse of cleansing friends.

Your life requires you to eat out more than once a week, travel a lot, and live without an eating schedule: You hopefully have at least 24 hours a week you can call your own. Make that your One-Day Reboot Cleanse.

You love, love, love meat: Begin with a Three-Day Blast to confirm that you can live without your daily visits to the butcher. Then consider a longer-term plan by implementing a regular schedule of Two-Week Full-Body Cleanses to counteract your usual saturated eating plan. Chances are you'll begin to eat less and less meat and find the same satisfaction from more healthy proteins, like nuts.

You smoke: Hopefully kicking ash is one of your New Year's resolutions. In the meantime, begin with a One-Day Reboot Cleanse, move up to a Three-Day Blast, followed in a few months by a Five-Day Fine-Tune, and finish the year with a Two-Week Full-Body Cleanse. Easing yourself into a no-smoke zone is easier and more geared for success if you take baby steps.

Your family is going to cleanse with you: If none or even one of you has never cleansed before, keep it short and sweet to ensure success. Aim for the Three-Day Blast but be prepared to tweak that down if you're hearing a lot of complaints, or it's guaranteed the next cleanse you do will be alone.

You're not really a big fruit and vegetable eater: Start with a One-Day Reboot Cleanse and work your way up to longer cleanses to slowly get used to what will be your new favorite (honest!) food group.

Your high school reunion is coming up and you seriously want to fit into your old school sweater: Block out 14 days and make sure your green smoothies don't have a lot of high-calorie add-ins. To lose one pound, you need to consume 3,500 fewer calories. Experts recommend that you eat 500 to 1,000 fewer calories each day depending on your current weight and how many pounds you want to lose. At this pace, you can lose 1 to 2 pounds of body fat per week (500 fewer calories per day x 7 days per week = 3,500 calories = 1 pound per week).

You have been eating life in the fast/processed-food lane: Give your body a break from digesting junk with a Five-Day Fine-Tune.

You need a quick feel-good boost: A One-Day Reboot Cleanse will leave you feeling lighter and brighter.

You don't want to tie up your weekend: Opt for a Monday through Friday Five-Day Fine-Tune.

You're the type of person who eats one slice of bread and it goes down your throat and directly on to your bottom: As long as you continue with a healthier eating plan once the cleanse is over, the Three-Day Blast will help your body start to process what it eats.

You know what whole foods are, and you have seen people buying them but you're too busy to deal with new foods: The One-Day Reboot Cleanse limits you to a few ingredients, making it actually easier to stick to than your regular diet.

You're "so" getting your full nutritional intake: Do you "cover your food groups" with things like salsa ("tomatoes"), potato chips ("potatoes"), pizza ("tomatoes," "grains," and "protein"), enriched breakfast cereal ("grains" and "daily vitamins"), and processed peanut butter ("protein")? You'll need to wean yourself off of the high-sodium and sugar-flavor fest, so try a Two-Week Full-Body Cleanse and incorporate lots of natural flavors that mimic the artificial ones you've been living on, like seaweed (salty), olive oil (healthy fat), and mango and apple (better sugars).

Cleansing Issues

Sometimes you want to go on a green smoothie cleanse because you feel subpar or you know you have been living the unwholesome life and want to get back in the green. Other times, your body is letting you know—loud and clear. Green smoothies are designed to make you feel better, long-term. So if you're experiencing any of the following, clear your calendar for a cleanse as soon as possible (while a Three-Day Blast or Five-Day Fine-Tune are optimal, even a One-Day Reboot Cleanse can kick-start you to feeling better):

- You have, ahem, issues with bloating, gas, burping, indigestion, constipation, diarrhea, or other digestive disorders.
- You often feel rundown or tired, no matter how much caffeine, soda, or energy drinks you gulp every hour.
- You have tried counting everything from sheep to memorizing the periodic table, but you still have difficulty falling asleep, staying asleep, or having a restful sleep.
- You feel like you're on a high wire and barely staying balanced.
- Your friends and family use words like "stress," "depression," "anxiety," and "mood swings" around you and send you articles about the benefits of antidepressants.
- The food in your kitchen seems to come from just one of these four groups: sugar, refined carbohydrates, junk food, or stimulants.
- You're constantly hungry, no matter how much you eat.

It's Okay to Fail

A green smoothie cleanse isn't just about powering through a set number of days in order to come out the other side a new, improved you. That's just the by-product. What cleansing is really all about is tuning in to your nutritional needs.

So remember to respect and listen to your body. It will tell you if something is wrong. It could be that you're experiencing, without relent, constant aches and pain or that you have just felt generally unwell from the get-go of your cleanse. Or maybe you felt on top of the world initially but now, after a few days of cleansing, you're feeling so poorly that catching the flu would seem like a tea party by comparison.

Fine. It happens. A cleanse shouldn't be something that you suffer through or tolerate (although there will be some of that, of course). It's also a chance to be present in your body and cleanse your inner self, too, to peel off the unnecessary in your life, both literally and metaphorically, that plagues you daily. Think of it as not only cleansing your digestive system and diet, but releasing contaminated emotions and feelings as well.

So if you're feeling so dreadful that you can't even think about, let alone drink, another green smoothie without gagging, don't beat yourself up. Give yourself permission to stop cleansing. There's no point in continuing if you're going to be miserable the entire time. Pick yourself up and try again later.

Another wake-up call is hunger that won't go away. The last thing you want is to be thinking compulsively about spaghetti Alfredo for the next however many days, which is probably what would have happened.

There is always the possibility that your body isn't in the mood to cleanse right now. It doesn't mean you should never have a green smoothie again or shouldn't try a green smoothie cleanse for the rest of your life. It means that right now isn't your time and next week or month might be.

THE BIG FAIL—AND HOW NOT TO BAIL

It's official. You didn't make it. Maybe you lasted an hour, a day, or even a week. But somewhere along the way, you craved and caved before your cleanse was over. What started out as a challenge to see if you could live on green smoothies for (insert the cleanse time length you chose) days ended up to be exactly that—a challenge. While a green smoothie cleanse—or any cleanse, for that matter—isn't necessarily the health answer for everyone (otherwise why would there be so many different kinds of healthy eating plans?), it isn't something you can really decide until you give it a fair shot. Green smoothie cleanses aren't like airline reward miles; you don't collect more points the longer you cleanse. This is about having the awareness that you need a change and the intent to make those changes. So you still get an A for effort. Plan on cleansing again, but first think about what made you buckle under. Here are some common cleanse setbacks and how to advance beyond them next time:

You focused on what you couldn't have rather than what you could: You felt that you couldn't go on any dates or out with friends, driving by your local junk food joint gave you pangs of deprivation (even though you don't really like fast food), you practically salivated at the thought of tearing into something edible with your teeth, you didn't feel the trade off of green leafy vegetables and fruit for fried food was worth it...Next time, try a shorter cleanse, even if it means half a day. Accomplishing your goal can make sticking to a healthier menu more palatable.

The taste of the green smoothie was not quite the delicious blend you had hoped for: Play with your ingredients. It's going to take a few tries to find your favorite flavor combos. And in the meantime, just suck it up, buttercup. You're so much tougher than 16 ounces of vegetable matter.

Your hunger pangs weren't as delayed as you had hoped: If you're really starving, then add another green smoothie to your daily menu. Sticking with the general plan is better than giving up altogether and inhaling a plate o' bad calories.

You couldn't take the migraines from the lack of coffee: Add some chicory to your green smoothie. It's an all-natural, caffeine-free coffee substitute. You'll need the root, where most of the kick is. If you can't find it fresh, check out a coffee store for roasted chicory root nibs or look for chicory root tea.

You thought, "One tiny triangle of nachos. Just one. No one will know": Which turned into two nachos, then a small mound, which you washed down with a beer and at that point, what the hell, a slice of mud pie: OK, so you "cheated." Big whoop. It happens. Don't make one slip up an excuse to stop altogether.

You were bored with your green smoothie: Insider secret: Variety is the spice of cleansing. Keep things interesting by regularly changing up your ingredients.

You dropped the weight you wanted to lose and began feeling really confident: So confident that you thought, "I have a handle on this cleansing thing—a little glass of wine/a taste of that cake/dinner out won't hurt, I can make up for it later." But later becomes never and you feel too depressed to start again: Plan to get back to basics with a One-Day Reboot Cleanse to re-prove to yourself that you can do it!

CHAPTER TEN

Prepping for the Program

While a green smoothie cleanse can certainly be used as a short-term fix for eating and drinking on the wild side (or planning to do so), the long-term plan is to create a healthier eating and living program for yourself. So however long you decide to cleanse, you'll need to do some planning beyond making sure you have access to fresh produce and a working blender and hiding the cookies. You're going to need to make some time for prepping pre-cleanse and transitioning post-cleanse.

That's right: prepare, prepare, prepare. The more prepared you are, the smoother your green smoothie cleanse will be.

The rule of thumb is to double the number of days you're cleansing—half for before and half for after. So if you're on a One-Day Reboot Cleanse, you'll need half day to ease into the cleanse and half a day to ease out of it; a Three-Day Blast will require six days altogether, an additional day and a half before and day and a half after, and so on. This is a minimum recommendation, since the longer you spend easing your mind and body in and out of cleansing mode, the easier, more comfortable, and more successful overall the entire experience is going to be (the people who suffer most through a cleanse, complaining of headaches, fatigue, nausea, and even vomiting, are usually the ones who dove right in after an eating and/or drinking frenzy).

The checklist below covers everything you need to get prepped for your green smoothie cleanse.

Prep Step One: Get Your Mind in the Mood

Before you can cleanse your body, you need to cleanse your mind. You don't want to start the cleanse all frazzled and stressed out. Use your pre-smoothie time to start a 15-minute de-stressing meditation.

- Accept this truth: Once you make the definite decision to cleanse, you'll begin to think in a Paleolithic way and become entirely consumed by food—gathering it, blending it, taking in calories.

- Expect weird cravings like anchovy ice cream. Missing ultrasalty and/or -sweet foods comes with the cleansing territory. Try and ride it out. Your hankerings, along with desires for the three C's (cigarettes, caffeine, and the main ingredient of cocktails) diminishes the longer you cleanse.

- Write down your cleanse mission statement; do this each and every time and for each and every kind of cleanse that you do. Think about the what's—what this cleanse means to you, what your immediate aims are, and what you hope to accomplish in the long-term. Keep this with you throughout your cleanse as your pocket reminder to help keep your goals in sight and your spirit strong. Taking the time to write down why you're cleansing and what you're hoping to achieve clarifies the mind and helps to motivate you to psych yourself into staying the course when you have a down, what's-it-all-about moment (which you definitely will).

- In addition, channel your inner sixth-grade girl and start keeping a cleansing journal before the cleanse begins. This is where you can write down your biggest fears (like you'll starve to death), your craziest hopes (that you'll lose 25 pounds on a one-day cleanse, for instance) and everything in between. Once you start cleansing, make a daily note of how you feel mentally and physically, how you slept, your energy levels throughout the day, your weight, and your reflections. Read through it the next time you're preparing for a cleanse for insight on what smoothie recipes worked for you in terms of energy, taste, and satisfaction (you might forget that you really did not like the texture of egg in a green smoothie or that a smoothie made with pineapple did not give you the morning energy boost you needed) and also timing (perhaps you prefer more fruit in your smoothie first thing in the morning or as a nightcap).

- Think out your schedule. Even if you have cleansed before, each time is different and you just don't know how you're going to react or deal. So while you do want to stay busy (to distract you from food cravings), try to avoid important meetings, stressful deadlines, big social events, and situations in which food has a starring role.

- Find a phone-a-cleansing-friend. Having someone who won't just give you support, but is also going through what you are will make your cleansing experience not just easier, but more fun. But be careful who you choose; someone may be your BFF but they may also be a slacker whose closest acquaintance with the word "finish" is that Finnish vodka they like to drink. Better to team up with a health-conscious, goal-oriented friend, family member, or coworker who will help you reach your goal. If there are a few of you, set a date midcleanse for a green smoothie cleansing party; think recipe exchanges, cups brimming with freshly blended green smoothie "cosmos," and a green smoothie challenge: Set up a blender, bowls of fruit and vegetables, pitchers of liquid, and containers with add-ins, and see who can come up with the best green smoothie combo (winnings can be a copy of this book!).

- Don't be a secret cleanser. Let your nearest and dearest and anyone you normally break bread with know that you're cleansing and that you would appreciate their support. Ideally they will support you; at the very least, they hopefully won't leave empty chip bags laying around. If you need some additional support, log on—there's a constant community of Greensters blogging about their experiences and standing by to shore you up, suggest recipes and tips for success, and sing the praises of green smoothie cleanses.

- Along the same lines, if you end up being a lone-cleanser, still plan on staying social. Even pre-cleanse, you may not feel like surrounding yourself with people. But there's something to be said for the group mentality and peer pressure. Seek your own kind, because once you start cleansing and reaping the benefits, you're going to sound like an infomercial pitchman for green smoothies. If no one you know is currently cleansing or has ever cleansed, find that online community. (As an added incentive, studies show that one of the nine shared traits of places on earth where people live the longest is a strong social network.)

- Don't expect quick results. Green smoothie cleanses aren't about instant gratification. You'll feel less than absolutely fabulous at first. But stick with it and you'll feel not just good, but better than you have ever felt before.

- With all of the above, remember: This isn't about no pain, no gain. A green smoothie cleanse is something you're doing *for* yourself, not *to* yourself (repeat as necessary).

Prep Step Two: Get Your Body in the Swing

Plan on building some siesta time into your schedule, such as your afternoon snack or caffeine break. Fogginess, grogginess, and touchiness are all initial downside symptoms of cleansing. Studies show that a regular practice of 20 to 90 minutes of power napping improves memory, motivation, and mood.

Get in the habit of getting off your butt. In reality. If most of your day consists of you being tethered to a desk, start taking a daily stand and get up and move around for a few minutes every hour or so. Sitting all day at work can be deadly in the long-term, even if you exercise regularly. When you're on a green smoothie cleanse, it can set you up for total exhaustion before the day has barely begun. The onset of a green smoothie cleanse isn't the time to begin an intense workout regimen. But if you already have a regular routine, don't stop because you're about to cleanse. Getting your heart pumping will help up flagging energy levels. If your favorite exercise to date has been lifting your legs to the coffee table while vegging out in front of the TV, then simply getting off the couch and walking will give you a boost. To keep moving during your cleanse and after, plan on clutching an ice cold green smoothie between your hot little palms. Research has found that people who touched a cold object to their palms when they were about to give up were able to work out longer than those who did not cool their hands.

Listen to your body to know when it's time to (re)cleanse (but limit yourself to four big cleanses a year). Some signs include constipation, congestion, sugar cravings, skin problems, temperature sensitivity, insomnia, and constant sniffles.

Prep Step Three:
Get Your Diet in the Groove

The idea of pre-cleansing your diet to get it ready for a cleanse seems out of whack. But the hard truth is that even if you're planning a quickie with a One-Day Reboot Cleanse, your long-term success rate is going to be much higher if you prep your eating plan. Gradually weaning yourself off of these oral crutches is definitely an easier option than going cold turkey:

Coffee and black tea: A cup a day pre-cleanse is fine if it's what you need to get you through the day without a caffeine withdrawal headache. Five cups, not so much. Pharmacologically, caffeine, like cigarettes, has addictive ingredients that could classify it as a drug. One fool-your-body tactic is to have a half-'n'-half—50 percent leaded and 50 percent unleaded—the first pre-cleanse day. Gradually rebalance the ratio until you have completely eliminated the caffeine. If you're missing the acidic flavor of coffee, a caffeine-free herbal coffee substitute such as Roastaroma tea might appease your taste-buds. Tea drinkers can switch and bait with ultralow-caffinated green, white, matcha, or oolong tea.

Liquor: Some people start raising their glasses like it's a new Olympic event pre-cleanse. This isn't a good idea. The effects of alcohol take a long time to wear off—possibly even longer than your cleanse—and are even worse if you already have liver or nutrition problems.

Cigarettes: You really need an explanation? Putting aside the cancer connection, cigarettes are truly toxic. They are stuffed with hazardous chemicals along the lines of pesticides, formaldehyde, vinyl chlorides, radioactive metals, arsenic, ammonia, carbon monoxide, hydrogen cyanide, and 4,000 other nasty ingredients. If that isn't enough to make you boot the butt, ponder this: While even one single cigarette can have serious adverse consequences on your body (including hardening of the arteries by a whopping 25 percent), all it takes is 20 minutes since your last cigarette for your body to begin healing itself. In addition, the longer you go without, the greater the positive effects.

Processed Foods: You can (try) to read the label and ditch anything with ingredients you don't know let alone can't pronounce. But much easier is to follow this simple rule from food activist and journalist Michael Pollan: If it isn't something Great-Granny ate, eliminate!

Salt: Sodium is worth a special mention because it's often hidden in the most unlikely places, including white bread, many breakfast cereals, jarred spaghetti sauce, canned vegetables, flavored rice, salad dressings, cottage and American cheese, and ketchup.

Plan your menu for the week and make time to grocery shop. Make room by ridding your life of any foods or beverages that might tempt you during your cleanse.

It should go without saying that you must continue taking your meds even during your cleanse, but it can't: Don't stop taking any prescription medications while on a green smoothie cleanse or any dietary elimination plan.

GIVE YOUR DIET A MINI-MAKEOVER

Many people adopt a "condemned prisoner's last meal" attitude and use the buildup days to their cleanse to overload on soon-to-be forbidden fare like steak and a martini. Those are the same people who start complaining of belly aches, fatigue, and headaches 15 minutes into their official green smoothie cleanse. The earlier you start eating clean, the smoother the actual cleanse experience will be. Here are five simple steps to cleaning your plate:

Step 1: Start drinking a green smoothie daily.

Step 2: Slowly up your daily fiber intake or the sudden influx when you make the switch to all green smoothies all the time may cause a sudden outpouring. Also, drink more water to accommodate your increased fiber intake to reduce indigestion.

Don't incorporate all of the following at once. Moderation is always the key in all things green smoothie. A large increase in fiber over a short period of time could result in abdominal problems such as bloating, diarrhea, gas, and all-around discomfort. Aim for three weeks to gradually include the following six high-and-easy fiber foods once a day:

1. Buy orange juice with pulp. Or better yet, just eat the oranges whole.

2. Put your vegetable peeler away. Almost all of the foods with a skin or a peel will probably have more fiber if you're eating that skin than if you're peeling it off. The easiest skins to eat are apple, potato, and cucumber.

3. Make a vow never to buy white bread again. Seriously. The flour that white bread is made from probably contains some nutrients, particularly the enriched varieties, but it lacks the nutritional punch or fiber you'll find in whole grain breads. "Flour, white flour, wheat flour, and plain flour" are all synonymous in the FDA's eyes. But while the FDA does not differentiate, you should. So memorize the following:

   - *Wheat flour* is made from grinding the entire wheat grain.
   - *White flour* is made from the endosperm only, which is the starchy protein part.
   - *Whole-grain* or *Whole-meal* flour is made from grinding the bran, endosperm, and germ.
   - *Wheat germ flour* is made from the endosperm and germ.

Food Swap

DON'T EAT	EAT THIS INSTEAD
Whole milk	Skim milk
White flour	Whole wheat flour
Enriched pasta	Whole-grain pasta
White rice	Brown or wild rice
Processed cereal	Oatmeal or any cooked whole grain
Soda	Water
Sour cream or mayonnaise	Plain yogurt or avocado
Butter	Olive oil or applesauce
White potatoes	Sweet potatoes
Croutons	Walnuts
Cream cheese	Almond butter
Sugar	Honey or maple syrup
Fruit juice	Whole Fruit
Veggie chips	Veggies

4. Snack on almonds. Many nuts are high in fiber but almonds win the Olympic gold.

5. Beans aren't just good for your heart. Legumes are one of the richest sources of fiber. Plus, you can easily add them to just about any meal: heated as a side, added to soups, chili, or salads, or served in place of meat as a main dish.

6. Leave the sugary cereals on the shelves, even if they boast that they have added fiber. Whole-grain cereals and bran flakes are just as easy to swallow and are full of fiber.

Step 3: Lose the processed sugar and fatty foods. Instead, pile your plate pre-cleanse with similar kinds of provisions that you'll be blending and drinking in a few days—fresh veggies, tofu, fruits, seeds, and lean meats like poultry or forage fish like sardines and mackerel.

Step 4: Plan—literally, make a reminder note—to eat a small pure food snack every couple of hours to stabilize blood sugar and your energy levels. Raw, unsalted almonds are the perfect pre–green smoothie cleanse snack because they are packed with filling fiber and protein and can easily make the switchover to a green smoothie add-in.

Step 5: Pour in the water. Water is the essence of any cleanse. Your body needs H_2O to function at peak efficiency. The cleanses in this book suggest a minimum water level, but you can certainly drink much, much more. Water will help to keep you feeling flushed and full, an important consideration as you cut out your favorite in-between meal fillers. You can squeeze a spritz of fresh lemon or lime or add some refreshing herbs like parsley or mint to the water to give it a fancy flare.

However, as with all drinking, knock back the H_2O smartly. There's no RDA for water or liquid consumption in general because how much each person needs to be hydrated each day is completely individual, depending on their size, weight, family history, health, fitness, perspiration levels, where they live, how hot it is, personal acclimatization to that environment, and recent degree of activity.

You can see why it's hard to measure. Still, know that you can get too wet. An overflow of any fluid can lead to hyponatremia, which is a water toxicity that occurs when sodium in the blood becomes too diluted. Here's how to sponge up without springing a leak:

- Do the urine test. Your first urine of the day should be copious and pale or clear. The rest of the day, your urine should continue to be mostly clear or close to lemonade. If it's more like iced tea, you're dehydrated.

- Avoid being thirsty. This isn't actually a good indicator because by the time the brain sends its signal for a fill up, your body's fluids are already depleted. Here, in depleting amounts, is how water flows through the body: 1) Urine, 2) Sweat, 3) Evaporation (other than sweat), and 4) Metabolic processes (water used inside the body) and respiration (water lost while exhaling). Both are negligible amounts compared with the first three.

Water Flavorings

Let's face it. While water is thirst-quenching, refreshing, and the kind of ingredient that gives nutritionists happy dreams, it can taste…well, that's the problem. It doesn't really taste like anything. Which is why flavored drinks and sodas are so popular. But you can dress up your H_2O to happy hour standard. Try chopping, slicing and/or dicing one or more of the following into your long, tall, cool drink of water. Each amount equals one Water Flavorings measure in the cleanse shopping lists.

- Vegetables (½ cup per pint of water) such as cucumbers, celery, beets, carrots
- Fruit (½ cup per pint of water) such as peaches, berries, melons, pears, mangoes
- Herbs (¼ cup per pint of water) such as mint, lemongrass, parsley, sage, ginger, basil
- Citrus (¼ fruit per pint of water) such as orange, pineapple, grapefruit, lemon, lime
- Baking extracts (1 teaspoon per pint of water) such as vanilla, almond, coconut

- Keep your body healthfully soaked by drinking in moderation throughout the day. And if you're thirsty, drink a little more than you need to drench yourself. Research shows that people underestimate the amount of fluid they need to rehydrate.
- Space out how often you swig back and never drink so much water that you feel physically full. This is overkill, and the full feeling is your body telling you so. Hyponatremia is more

likely to occur when large amounts are consumed in a short period of time. As long as you're spreading out your sips throughout the day, your kidneys should be able to handle and filter the water. A good watermark is 16 ounces every couple of hours as long as you're also urinating every couple of hours. If you're exercising, increase that to 8 ounces of water for every 20 minutes of exercise.

- All fluids count—even tea. All teas, including green, are mild diuretics. But the amount is so minuscule that it won't have a dehydrating effect.

Prep Step Four: Get Yourself in the Know

Know that the Scouts are right—you must be prepared. So even though the time you're going to end up investing overall in your green smoothie cleanse is going to be longer than the actual cleanse itself, it's important to make room in your schedule for the pre-cleanse prep and post-cleanse transition.

Know that a cleanse isn't the same thing as a fast. This cannot be stated too much. A fast is just a faddy way of starving the body. This isn't healthy and is unlikely to be successful at anything other than making you stressed and sluggish. The body is evolutionarily hard-wired to combat starvation (prolonged fasting) by going into self-preservation autopilot once the food stops coming in. It slows down metabolism and increases the production of cortisol, which goes to work breaking down muscle tissue in order to liberate certain amino acids (proteins) that can be converted to sugar to feed the brain, red blood cells, and kidneys. When you go on a green smoothie cleanse, you'll be feeding your body plenty of nutrients and enough calories to keep it from switching into panic mode. It's designed to simply help your body do what it does best: cleanse and detoxify itself naturally.

Know that your start date can affect your success, even if you're doing a One-Day Reboot Cleanse. For instance, it may be easier to begin your cleanse on a non-work day because you can completely focus on the task of cleansing. Or, you may prefer to blend on a work day because you'll have other things grabbing your attention or you feel the routine will make it easier for you to stick to the cleansing plan.

Know your menstrual cycle (if you're a woman). If you have a tough period with heavy bleeding and painful cramps, you have enough going on without having to deal with the challenges that can come with being on a cleanse. However, once you're in a cleansing rhythm, you may find that your pesky periods have become a lot more manageable in which case, cleanse away.

Know that you should always clear a cleanse with your doctor if you're pregnant or nursing (if you're a woman). It's generally not considered a good idea to go a on cleanse regimen while a growing baby is dependent on your body for its calories.

Know that life throws more curves than a Victoria's Secret model's body. So if an unexpected invite like dinner with out-of-town friends or drinks with the boss suddenly lands in your in-box when you're just about to embark or are mid-cleanse, it's perfectly OK to switch-hit to a shorter cleanse this time. This is about making you feel better, not guilty.

Know too that if, at any point, your body is saying, "This is way too intense. Seriously. This isn't about missing food. I feel really sick!" then stop the cleanse immediately and plan on picking it up at a later date. This is about making you feel good about yourself and your diet. If it's making you feel sicker than a goldfish out of water, then your cleanse isn't achieving its aims. Your reaction could be due to the green smoothies, but if you followed the prepping advice and tried a few without any reaction, it's more likely that this moment in time isn't the right one for you to be cleansing. You might be too stressed or feeling under the weather or simply in a non-cleansing state of mind. It happens. Try again in a few weeks (see It's OK to Fail, page 118).

Know that getting enough shut-eye will help you stick with the cleanse. Studies show that people who are chronically sleep-deprived may feel hungrier and have a yearning for high-carb foods (which are a quick source of energy). Aim for seven to nine hours of zzzz's per night.

Know that sleep is also vital to a successful cleanse. This isn't a repeat of the previous tip. A successful cleanse isn't about the length of cleanse time itself, but the long-term effect the cleanse has on your eating habits and lifestyle. When you cleanse, it's imprinted on your short-term memory, which is also known as the working, primary, active memory. These memories have a very short shelf life. In order to make a lasting impression, the effects of the cleanse need to be imprinted on the long-term memory, which is a permanent storage area. Part of the process of turning fleeting short-term memories into lasting long-term memories occurs when we are grabbing some shut-eye. Initial research suggests around eight hours ought to hardwire your brain into thinking about a healthier diet.

Know that a green smoothie cleanse, no matter how many days, is just that—green smoothies. However, if you feel that if you don't munch some food within the next 30 minutes, you may succumb to gnawing off your arm, just make a meal of the same exact foods (in the same exact measurements) as your green smoothie. Keep everything raw if possible and make like a cow and chew each bite until it's fully chomped.

Know that you should drink the rainbow. Yes, the name of the smoothie is "green" but we need a full rainbow of fruit and vegetable colors to reap the benefits of those nine required servings. There are unique phytochemicals, or plant chemicals, that vary from color to color. These various compounds all do different things to protect your health. So stick with the leafy green base but add a variety of red, white, purple/blue, and yellow/orange hues.

Know that your green smoothie can become the caloric equivalent of downing a soda if you super-stack it with add-ins. A classic 16-ounce green smoothie with just water, greens and fruit will usually weigh in under 400 calories. But one loaded up with calorie-dense foods like bananas, chocolate, mangoes, red grapes, goji berries, sweet potato, oats, hemp seeds, coconut, or dates can easily climb to 1,000-plus calories! Unless you're trying to gain weight, less is more.

Know that however satisfied, satiated, strong, and smiling you feel on your cleanse, there will be a moment—usually within the first few hours and then again, with more vigor, on day three (see below for more in the know tips on getting through the third day)—when you'll feel tempted to stray. Make your life easier by removing all lures from your vision line: Ditch the junk food, avoid after-work drinks with friends, whatever you need to do to get through the slump and finish clean.

Know that once you get past that desire to cheat, it often becomes irrelevant. You may actually swing in the opposite direction where you now have the yen to cleanse forever.

Know that however fantastic your cleanse makes you feel, the saying "too much of a good thing holds" true here. Follow the recommended cleansing schedule and don't over-cleanse. It won't kill you, but there really isn't any health benefit to depriving yourself from chewing a (healthy) plate of food.

Know that you're probably not going to smack your lips in delight after your first taste of a green smoothie. It's an acquired tasted—and one certainly worth acquiring. If you really find it unpalatable, try playing with your ingredients: use a milder leafy green such as spinach, add a sweeter fruit such as mango or one with a stronger taste such as pineapple, or, if it's the texture that is making you wrinkle your nose, give it a creamier base with a dollop of yogurt or an overripe banana. It usually only takes a couple of smoothies to adjust.

Know that you may feel uncomfortable and possibly even want to hurl hours after drinking the first smoothie of your cleanse. The less that greens (mostly) and fruit were a part of your daily life before cleansing, the worse you're probably going to feel. You could push through and thin your smoothies with more water or ice cubes to help with the gagging. This will probably help stop you from having a wretched retch reaction. But if the idea of even blending up another smoothie is making you gag, then crank it back. Forget the cleanse for now and instead, just try to acclimatize yourself to drinking a green smoothie a day and also include more whole vegetables, fruits, and protein in your regular diet. You'll still reap some of the benefits and be more willing to try a cleanse again in six months or so.

Know that you may initially feel famished on your cleanse. Add some protein to give your body a fully satisfied feeling. If your hunger is accompanied by a headache, skip the ibuprofun. Instead, try drinking more water. Other easy-on-the-stomach natural remedies include wearing a headband and rubbing peppermint oil on your temples.

Know, however, that you probably only think you're hungry. Honest. We don't really need to eat as much as we think. Our society today has oversold the need for a huge meal. After a few days on the green smoothie cleanse, you begin to realize that a lot of your daily eating is due to socializing, boredom, or simply because the food is there.

Know that the third day of a long-term cleanse is the hardest day. This is when you start to break down and people will start to look like walking French fries. Don't think long-term, as in, "I have X days left of this cleanse and I will never make it!" Focus instead on the next five minutes. And five minutes after that. And so on until you get through the slump. Most people start feeling fantastic by the fourth day.

Know that a green smoothie cleanse isn't just about what you do and don't put into your body. It's about what you do with your new feel-fantastic self. The more you make time to keep your body moving while cleansing, the better you will ultimately feel. How much you exercise depends on you and what you're already used to. Obviously, this isn't the time to finally start training for that marathon you have been meaning to run, but if you're used to a good sweat, then go ahead and perspire. If a walk or a morning salute to the sun is more your thing, then continue with that program. But at all times, listen to your body. If you feel too tired or achy to do what you usually do, then cut back by half and continue cutting until you reach a place that feels comfortable.

Know that if you have a fast food habit, it's worth taking a field trip to your favorite joint midway through a multiple-day cleanse. There are few things less appealing than the sight and smell of junk meat when you're on a purifying high. Chances are you'll lose your taste for the drive-through meal permanently.

Know that gas is a side effect of a diet of green smoothies. Everything in food has to be broken down into small bits in order to enter the bloodstream. Protein must be broken into its individual amino acids, fats must be broken into fatty acids, and carbohydrates (both simple and complex) must be broken into individual glucose (or equivalent) molecules.

Flatulence occurs when a food does not break down completely in the stomach and small intestine. As a result, the food makes it into the large intestine in an undigested state. The reality of a green smoothie is that no matter how much you blend or how super-powered your blender, there will always be a little something left to get your teeth into. So one way to cut down on the bottom burps is to chew your sips of drink. Think of it this way: Digestion begins in the mouth. If you're still tooting, limit starchy veggies and legumes and high-sorbitol fruit such as apples, beets, broccoli, Brussels sprouts, cabbage, carrots, cauliflower, corn, eggplant, green beans, peaches, pears, peas, prunes, pumpkin, squash, and zucchini, which are all hard on your digestive system.

Know that by the second day of any cleanse, you may as well have all your calls forwarded to the toilet because that is where you'll be spending a lot of time (something to factor in if you're going on a long journey). One of the side effects of cleansing is peeing and pooping…often (read: sometimes as much as once an hour initially).

Know that while you're in the toilet, you'll become obsessed with your poop. This means its texture (looser), its color (green), and its frequency (often). Know that no one else will be interested unless they too are on a cleanse.

Mega doses of certain fruits and veggies can have a Technicolor or fragrant effect on your bodily emissions.

IF THE HUE OF YOUR STOOL IS:	IT MIGHT BE CAUSED BY:
Purple	Beets
Red	Beets, tomato juice
Maroon	Tomato juice
Black	Blueberries
Orange	Carrots, sweet potatoes, kale, spinach, turnip greens, winter squash, collard greens, cilantro, thyme
Yellow	Carrots, sweet potatoes
Green	Green leafy vegetables

IF THE HUE OF YOUR URINE IS:	IT MIGHT BE CAUSED BY:
Pink	Beets, blackberries, rhubarb
Red	Beets, blackberries, rhubarb
Dark brown/tea colored	Rhubarb, fava beans, aloe
Orange	Carrots, carrot juice, vitamin C
Fluorescent yellow-green	B vitamins
Green (with sulphurish odor)	Asparagus

If the rainbow excrement or stinky pee continue once your cleanse is over, you should get it checked out, as it might be a sign of a more serious problem with your digestive system.

Know going back on solids is going to cause a big bowel evacuation. However, the diet change can make those movements painful. You can take the sting out by continuing to eat many of the foods in your smoothie recipe—drink lots of water, eat whole high-fiber fruits and veggies like apricots, papaya, peaches, pears, pineapples, prunes, legumes, greens, asparagus, broccoli, squash, and Brussels sprouts, and whole-grain foods.

Know that if you're a meat eater, it's better to return to your carnivore diet Asian-style. In other words, add tiny pieces of meat gradually rather than sitting down to a steak dinner the day after you finish your cleanse. Your stomach and heart will thank you for your reserve.

Know that after your cleanse, you're going to feel Frosted Flakes grrrreat! Lighter in spirit, mind, and body, and your complexion will look model-shoot fantastic.

CHAPTER ELEVEN

Easing Back into Eating

There is no finish line. So don't dive headfirst into a feeding trough post-cleanse. In fact, skip the happy ending meal altogether. After your cleanse, you're hopefully going to feel better than you have ever felt before, with more energy, more mental clarity, more efficient digestion, more, more, more! But you'll soon lose that post-cleanse glow if you jump back into a diet filled with fatty, fried foods. Take it slow. Ease yourself back into solids, but continue to try and eat clean (see Good for Your Gut, page 146) and green and whip up a daily green smoothie. Think of it as the cleanse after the cleanse.

Understand your game plan. This isn't about dieting, which is unhealthy and usually unsuccessful because it isn't sustainable for the long-term. This is about clean, green eating. For life.

Stick to a simple menu plan. Eat only foods with ingredients you not only recognize and can pronounce, but know were not cooked up in a laboratory.

Keep it light and slow. During a cleanse, you're consuming much less than you usually do. Even though you were feeling full and satisfied while on the cleanse, as you transition off it, start with smaller-than-you-are-used-to-and-possibly-want portions and take your time to chew and appreciate the food's flavor and texture. Aim for three meals a day, each with a beginning and an end and, if you need them, two in-between healthy (which is not a cagey way of saying sugary, starchy, or saturated in oils) snacks. The best in-between meal filler is a green smoothie, but other diet-healthy ways to stop tummy grumbles include:

- A handful of dried fruit: Keep it healthy by making sure there's no added sugars.

- A handful of nuts: Keep it healthy by checking the salt content. Eat raw or opt for brands with 50 percent salt.

- A couple of tablespoons of nut butter: Keep it healthy by reading the label to make sure that there's no added sugar or oil or make your own (see Make It, Don't Buy It, page 82).

- Baked sweet potato chips: Keep it healthy by reading the label, as some baked chips are just as high as the fried kind in trans fats, added sugar, and/or sodium. You can make it yourself easily enough (thinly slice an unpeeled sweet potato, toss with 1 tablespoon of olive oil, season with your favorite flavorings such as salt, pepper, cinnamon, or cumin, and bake on a baking sheet in a 400°F oven for 20 minutes, flipping halfway, until crisp and golden) but it really only works well if you have a mandolin to get the right thickness of the chip.

- A piece of fresh fruit: Keep it healthy by opting for a banana, especially as a post-cleanse snack, as they are high in fiber, which helps to restore normal bowel function, as well as electrolytes and potassium that may be lost due to runny stool.

Diffuse your morning drink. Chugging a high-octane coffee or tea after time off has a bizarro effect of giving you the kind of jittery buzz you crash from. Start with 50 percent strength and limit yourself to one cup a day. You might gradually increase your perk intake, but try not to exceed two cups to avoid caffeine side effects such as insomnia, restlessness, irritability, upset stomach, rapid heartbeat, and muscle tremors.

Make a separate post-cleanse shopping list. This will help you stick your plan. To keep your diet clean, check the ingredients of all packaged foods; leave them on the shelf if:

- The first three ingredients are "sugar."
- They have any ingredient ending in "ose"—these are added sugars (the two exceptions are lactose and fructose).
- They have any ingredient ending in "ol"—these are sugar alcohols, which are fattening and can also lead to bloating and diarrhea.

Continue to guzzle water. Drinking some H_2O during and after meals aids digestion and keeps you off the hard stuff: sodas, juices, and sugary yogurt drinks. Also, a glass of water can help you stop snacking. If you're still hungry 15 minutes after your drink, then go ahead and choose an Eat This snack (page 146).

Break your daily fast. You've heard it said countless times that breakfast is important, and you'll hear it one time more here because over one-fifth of adults are morning food skippers because they don't feel hungry or think it's a good way to cut calories. Bad idea. Studies show that those same people tend to pack more weight than those who eat a well-balanced breakfast. This is because eating breakfast kick-starts your metabolism for the day and keeps it going strong throughout the morning. Also, passing over breakfast might leave you famished by lunch, causing you to overdo it to compensate. Add in that a morning meal gives you a better memory, better energy, better impulse control, better concentration, and better cholesterol levels, and it seems obvious that you definitely shouldn't give it a miss when you're cleansing. If you really can't stomach the idea of food first thing, then keep it small—blend up a green smoothie or eat a granola bar or a piece of fruit.

Know which fats are your friends. You need to consume some fat for your body to function correctly. However, it's important to choose the right kinds of fats. Most animal fats and some vegetable oils are high in the kind of fats that raise your LDL cholesterol levels, the bad cholesterol. However, monounsaturated fatty acids are good fats, and you want to try to eat these regularly. They help lower the bad cholesterol in your body by raising the good cholesterol. Foods that are high in monounsaturated fatty acids are olive oil, nuts, fish oil, and various seed oils. (Adding these "good" fats to your weekly diet can lower your cholesterol and reduce your risk of heart disease.) The kind of fat you want to reject like a vampire avoids garlic are trans fats. A form of unsaturated fat, these are commonly found in processed foods. Consuming them raises your risk of heart disease. Read the labels of what you eat, and look for "partially hydrogenated" anything on the ingredient list as a warning. Keep in mind that in the U.S., manufacturers are allowed to advertise 0g of trans fat if the actual content is less than 0.5g.

Don't skip the carbs. They are your body's prime source of energy. The skinny is to understand the difference between the different carbs. In a nutshell (nuts = complex carbs), simple carbohydrates are digested quickly, and complex carbs, which tend to contain more fiber, take more time. Simple carbohydrates are found naturally in fruit, milk, and table sugar, while foods that contain complex carbohydrates include beans, whole-grain breads, and starchy vegetables. Our bodies need both simple and complex carbs in moderation. What they do not need is refined carbs such as white flours, white rice, white pastas, white sugars, soft drinks, fruit juices, corn syrup, and candy. Refined carbs, whether they are complex or simple, are like toothless dragons—mostly useless but potentially dangerous.

Join the Meatless Monday Movement. You can do it any day of the week. The premise is that most of us already get enough animal meat in our diets, so once a week skip protein altogether or switch it out with legumes, beans, or tofu.

Post-Cleanse Sample Menu

Your best happily-ever-after day-to-day menu for eating yourself out of a cleanse. Think flexible, meaning you can shuffle one day's food meal or food plan with another, if that works best with your schedule:

Post One-Day Reboot Cleanse Sample Menu—Eat for one to two days:

Breakfast: Fruit and ¼ cup of yogurt or kefir

Lunch: Salad with nuts, whole grains, and one hard-boiled egg.

Dinner: Lightly steamed vegetables, miso soup with vegetables and tofu, or vegetable soup.

Post Three-Day Blast Cleanse Sample Menu:
Eat for two to three days:

Day 1: A few pieces of fruit, raw or lightly steamed vegetables, leafy green salad, 1 cup of cooked grains or brown rice.

Day 2: Follow Day 1 and add a bowl of yogurt or kefir.

Day 3: Follow Day 2 and add a maximum of two poached or boiled eggs and 4 ounces of either poached or baked white fish or roasted chicken.

Post Five-Day Fine-Tune Sample Menu
Follow the Post Three-Day Blast Sample Menu and add the following for one to two more days:

Day 4: Increase protein like eggs, fish, or chicken to 6 ounces.

Day 5: If desired, add 4 ounces of dairy.

Post Two-Week Full-Body Cleanse Sample Menu

Days 1 to 3: Eat only vegetables, fruits, nuts, seeds, lentils, plant-based oils, and seasonings.

Day 4: Introduce white fish, legumes, beans, and grains such as brown rice, quinoa, and oats; go easy on the salt.

Day 5: Add eggs and/or soy (such as tofu or edamame) to your menu.

GOOD FOR YOUR GUT

In theory, you can digest anything you put in your mouth—including dirt and gum—but that doesn't mean you should eat whatever comes to mind. Hopefully, your post-cleanse diet will reflect a greener, cleaner diet that is good for your digestion and therefore, good for you.

Eat This

Yogurt: Possibly the number-one probiotic food. Probiotics are "good bugs" your body needs that aid digestion and promote immunity. Around 4 pounds of our body weight comes from the good bacteria that live in the digestive tract.

> *Watch out for:* Yogurt that isn't listed as "live" or "active" or that is flavored with a lot of sugar, which actually feeds the bad bacteria that also lives in the GI tract.

Lean meat and fish: If you're going to eat meat, go for chicken, fish, and other lean meats—your gut can handle them much better than red meat, which tends to be fattier. And lean meats and fish have not been associated with an increased risk of colon cancer like high-fat red meats have.

> *Watch out for:* Luncheon meats. Roast turkey or chicken sounds like it fits the lean meat category, but luncheon meats tend to be processed and high in sodium, nitrates, and possibly saturated fats, putting them in the same high colon cancer risk category as sausages and hot dogs.

Canned herring, sardines, anchovies, and mackerel: It turns out that eating forage-type fish is better for the environment, a busy lifestyle, and the stomach. These fish are high in the omega-3 fatty oils that help dampen down the inflammatory response so the body isn't constantly producing clotting agents. This helps sufferers of stomach ulcers or anyone with an upset stomach from a high-acid diet.

> *Watch out for:* Canned foods are the original fast food. When choosing canned foods, opt for whole foods like water-packed fish, vege-

tables, legumes, and fruit and read the label to make sure they don't contain added sodium or sugar. Canned foods should be rinsed and drained before eating to keep the sodium down.

Water: Water is the most essential "food" of all. Digestion can't occur without water because it helps move things through the intestines.

Watch out for: Flavored and/or "vitamin" water. Water is a healthy, hydrating, and rejuvenating miracle elixir. These flavored waters are the equivalent of a sugary flat soda. See Water Flavorings, page 132, for how to cleanly add a savory or sweet sensation to your H_2O.

Lentils: Bacteria multiply very quickly but need food once they reach the intestines. Prebiotics like the kind found in lentils help good bacteria thrive while driving down the number of disease-producing bacteria trying to invade the digestive tract. They also encourage a more acidic intestinal environment, which helps the body absorb nutrients like the minerals calcium, iron, zinc, and magnesium in food.

Watch out for: Nothing! It's all good!

Fermented foods like kimchi: And cabbage is a type of fiber that's not digested, so it helps eliminate waste, keeping bowel movements regular. Sauerkraut is good for the same reasons. Fermented foods that have the superpower of making food more digestible by actually "predigesting" it are beneficial. In short, they give the GI tract a vacation. Pickles, kefir, miso, tempeh, soy sauce, sourdough bread, sauerkraut, and the Korean pickle kimchi are all popular fermented foods.

Watch out for: Sourdoughs made with white flour instead of whole wheat and the high sodium content in soy sauce (there are reduced-sodium versions available).

Not That

These foods really should be permanently off of your menu, but if you feel you cannot live without them, then reintroduce them very *slowly* to your diet post-cleanse.

Fried foods: The high fat content in donuts, fries, onion rings, lots of happy hour bar food, potato chips, and anything fried can overwhelm the stomach, resulting in acid reflux and heartburn.

Clue that you are high on the fry: Your stools will go from their cleanse-period vivid green to insipidly pale-colored. This phenomenon actually has a name—steatorrhea, which is essentially excess fat in the feces.

Fatty foods: These foods stimulate contractions in the digestive tract, which, surprisingly, can either slow down the emptying of the stomach and worsen constipation or speed up movement and lead to or worsen diarrhea. Either way, it isn't fun in the sun. The effect can depend on the type of fat and your tendency toward constipation or diarrhea. Eat small meals spaced throughout the day, which can put less pressure on your stomach.

Clue that you are getting too much fat: Like with fried foods, your stools turn an ugly 50 shades of gray.

Alcohol: Your mind isn't the only thing a couple of drinks unwinds; alcohol also relaxes the esophageal sphincter, which can lead to acid reflux or heartburn. Nutritionally speaking, alcohol is a big fat zero. It has no protein vitamins, other nutrients, or "good" carbs. In fact, alcohol is toxic to the stomach lining and certain enzymes, prevents nutrients from being absorbed, and changes liver metabolism.

Clue that you are drinking too much: You're having more than one (women) to two (men) drinks a day and/or indigestion.

Coffee, tea, and carbonated beverages with caffeine: These drinks may be your go-to to get through the day, but they over-relax the esophageal sphincter, which keeps stomach acid confined to the stomach, and stimulate gastrointestinal tract motility, making contents move more, sometimes too quickly through your system.

Clue that you are overcaffeinated: You have diarrhea and cramping and/or heartburn.

Chile peppers: This staple of spicy cuisine can irritate the esophagus and lead to heartburn pain.

Clue that you are overspiced: You're experiencing nausea, vomiting, and diarrhea.

Corn: Fiber-rich corn is good for you, but it also contains cellulose, a type of fiber that humans can't break down easily because we lack a necessary enzyme. Our evolutionary ancestors were probably able to break it down with bigger, stronger teeth. If you chew corn longer, you can probably digest it just fine. But that can make socializing at the neighborhood barbecue difficult.

Clue that you are getting too corny: It has passed through you undigested and you're experiencing gas and abdominal pain.

Tomatoes: This and other citrus fruits, such as lemons, limes, oranges, and grapefruits are acidic, so while their vitamin C content is good for you, they can cause digestive problems.

Clue that you are getting too much acid: Your stomach is often upset after eating or drinking.

Processed foods: You want to avoid these foods anyway, but that goes triple if you're constipated, because they lack fiber, which helps to regulate bowel movements, are high in sodium, which causes water retention, and are often high in trans fats, manmade fats that are modified vegetable-derived fat, which can irritate the digestive process. These foods also often contain preservatives and artificial coloring, so people with allergies or sensitivities to these additives will feel their effects during digestive problems.

Clue that you are getting too much trans fat: Your fridge is full of premade meals that just require you to press a microwave button to prepare.

Artificial sweeteners: Sorbitol is most often associated with digestive problems. It's a hard-to-digest sugar found naturally in some fruits, including prunes, apples, and peaches, and is also used to sweeten gum and diet foods. Once sorbitol reaches the large intestine, it often creates gas, bloating, and diarrhea.

Clue that you may be getting too much sorbitol: You have persistent diarrhea.

Chocolate: It's a tragedy, but chocolate is the culprit of many digestive problems, including heartburn and the more serious GERD (gastro-esophageal reflux disease).

Clue that you've been getting too much chocolate: It seems unlikely that you wouldn't know if you OD'd on chocolate, but if your stomach is upset after indulging, it's a sure sign you need to lay off.

Spoiled foods: Duh, obviously. Except that bacteria such as salmonella and E. coli can pass from raw meat to veggies and fruits without any signs of contamination.

Clues that you are being "poisoned" by your food: You regularly have an upset stomach or feel nauseous.

DIRTY WORDS

Clean eating post-cleanse means choosing food that is minimally processed. That means checking labels to make sure you're not eating these 13 little-known, flavor-enhancing, often lab-generated words:

I. Artificial Coloring: Food colorings make food into eye candy, but many have been linked with an array of cancers and possible disorders in children. The main culprits are Blue I and 2, Red 3, Green 3, and Yellow 6, but all are potentially unhealthy. Companies have begun removing dye from children's foods in Europe.

Popular foods containing these artificial colorings: salmon, beverages, candy, baked goods, pet food dye, cherries, fruit cocktail, sausage, gelatin, cheese, yogurt, and hundreds more.

2. Artificial and natural flavors: Natural flavors derive from nature, but not necessarily from what the label implies. For example, strawberry and vanilla flavor can come from the gland in a beaver's backside. Scientists manipulate the molecules to give the taste impression of something natural, like a papaya or a strawberry. Artificial flavorings also bear no relation to the real food flavor and are completely manmade from chemicals. These artificial flavors are often substituted for that food as a cheaper replacement and/or composed in a way to increase some foods' "more-ish" qualities, turning the eater into an addict.

Popular foods containing artificial flavors: Almost everything.

3. Artificial sweeteners: Turns out that these sugar substitutes aren't so sweet in the long run. Not only do they potentially cause you to consume more calories, their origins make them sound like a science experiment gone wrong.

- Sucralose: Chlorinated sugar. That's right—as in chlorine, as in bleach.

- Saccharin: This sweetener is made from a compound derived from petroleum. Although ruled safe by the FDA, there's a question over whether it contributes to cancerous cell growth.

- Aspartame: Made from a combination of two amino acids, there's a lot of controversy but no solid evidence regarding its health risks.

- Acesulfame-K: Also known as acesulfame potassium, one of the solvents used to make it is methylene chloride, which may have carcinogenic characteristics.

Popular foods containing artificial sweeteners: Currently used in more than 5,000 products around the world, including candies, table-top sweeteners, chewing gums, beverages, dessert and dairy product mixes, baked goods, alcoholic beverages, syrups, refrigerated and frozen desserts, and sweet sauces and toppings.

4. BHA (Butylated Hydroxyanisole) and BHT (Butylated Hydroxy-toluene): Turns out not all antioxidants are good for you. These antioxidant preservatives have been ID'd as known carcinogens by the Department of Health and Human Services and banned nearly world-wide, but the FDA still gives them the all clear. They have been shown to have a negative effect on sleep and appetite and are connected with liver and kidney damage, hair loss, behavioral problems, cancer, fetal abnormalities, and growth retardation.

Popular foods containing BHA or BHT: Breakfast cereals, potato chips, vegetable oils, baked products, many canned or frozen soups and stews, ice cream, gelatin desserts, dry mixes for desserts, unsmoked dry sausage, beer, pet food, and chewing gum.

5. Enriched wheat: A fancy way of saying that the niacin, thiamine, riboflavin, folic acid, and iron that naturally occur in wheat products were stripped out during the refining process and then added back in, but not in any way that will bring it back to its nutritionally worthy former self.

Popular foods containing enriched wheat: bread, flour, even wheat, rye, and other grains. An extra FYI—some flours are also bleached.

6. High-fructose corn syrup (aka the recently relabeled "corn sugar"): Chemically similar to table sugar (i.e., sucrose), this cheaper alternative is a highly processed form of glucose converted into fructose, the type of sugar ordinarily found in fruit. While there's no conclusive evidence as to its health risks, the real problem is that this highly-processed syrup is an added ingredient in a surprising number of food products that you wouldn't suspect contained sugar.

Popular foods containing high-fructose corn syrup: English muffins, rolls, white and whole wheat bread, pizza sauce, spaghetti sauce, ketchup, barbecue sauces, soft drinks, tonic, most breakfast cereals, fruit drinks, flavored water, lunch meats, dinner sausage, macaroni and cheese, many salad dressings, pretzels, yogurts, cocktail peanuts, preserves, applesauce, whipped cream, crackers, pickles, packaged stuffing, nutrition bars…get the picture?

7. MSG (Monosodium Glutamate): The original undercover additive, MSG goes by over 40 different aliases, including maltodextrin, sodium caseinate, textured protein, hydrolyzed pea protein, autolyzed yeast, autolyzed vegetable protein, hydrolyzed vegetable protein, yeast extract, and even citric acid and natural flavoring, making it difficult to recognize on the label. Whichever name it's going by, MSG has been linked with migraines, seizures, infections, abnormal neural development, certain endocrine disorders, specific types of obesity, and especially the neurodegenerative diseases, a group of diseases that includes ALS (Lou Gehrig's Disease), Parkinson's disease, Alzheimer's disease, Huntington's disease, and olivopontocerebellar degeneration.

Popular foods containing MSG: Chinese take-out, canned and instant soup, diet drinks, many fast foods, packaged sausages and frankfurters, beef stew, salad dressing, some packaged vegetarian foods, salty snack chips, soy sauce, luncheon meats, packaged gravy, dipping sauces, and chicken products (nuggets, tenders, sausage).

8. Partially hydrogenated oil: The number-one source for the nutritional evildoer trans fat. These fats are actually twice as tough for the body to dissolve as their almost-as-disreputable cousin, saturated fats. They also have an adverse effect on cholesterol, jacking up the bad (LDL) kind and lessening the good (HDL) kind, sending them to the top of the dietary list as a cause of heart disease, diabetes, nutritional deficiencies, and cellular deterioration. Don't get duped by a zero–trans fat boast—read the fine print. Food that contains partially hydroge-nated oils but has less than 0.5g of trans fat per serving can call them-selves "trans fat free." Also keep in mind that "fully hydrogenated oil" does not contain trans fats.

Popular foods containing trans fats: margarine, vegetable shortening, crackers, cookies, baked goods, salad dressings, breads, and chips.

9. Potassium benzoate: A food preservative that helps prevent the growth of mold, yeast, and some bacteria, it's also used as the sound agent in many fireworks. In the European Union, it isn't recommended for consumption by children.

Popular foods containing potassium benzoate: fruit juice, sparkling drinks, pickles, margarine, olives, apple cider, low-fat salad dressings, syr-ups, and jams. It's just as hazardous as sodium benzoate, so read your labels.

10. Potassium sorbate: Some people suffer from side effects from this preservative, including headaches, nausea, and diarrhea.

Popular foods containing potassium sorbate: wine, dried fruits, baked goods, ice cream, yogurt, and herbal supplements.

11. Propyl gallate: An antioxidant preservative often used in conjunc-tion with BHA and BHT to protect oils and fats in foods, cosmetics, hair products, adhesives, and lubricant products from oxidation, it has been possibly linked to cancer.

Popular foods containing propyl gallate: meat products, chicken soup base, and chewing gum.

12. Sodium nitrate and sodium nitrite: These preservative additives are also used in the production of fertilizers, pyrotechnics, glass, and solid rocket propellant. If that doesn't kill your appetite, they have been tied to Alzheimer's, diabetes mellitus, and Parkinson's disease, as well as gastric, colorectal, esophageal, and colon cancers.

Popular foods containing sodium nitrate and sodium nitrite: hot dogs, bacon, and sausage deli meats.

13. Sugar as the first or second ingredient: This is the single largest source of calories for Americans and is stuffed into foods it has no business being in.

Popular foods containing sugar: Deli meats, pretzels, cheese spread, fruit juices, infant formula, and many processed and/or packaged foods.

NINE FOODS YOU NEED TO BAN FROM YOUR LIFE RIGHT NOW

1. Butter-flavored microwave popcorn: The fake butter flavoring alone should be a giveaway. In addition, microwave popcorn's bag liner contains PFOA, a proven toxicant and carcinogen that clings to the popcorn when heated.

Skip the packaged microwave popcorn on movie night and put ¼ cup of corn kernels in a brown paper lunch bag, fold the top, pop it in the microwave, and drizzle with olive oil or a little butter. Cheap, easy, and MacGyver-worthy.

2. Deli meats: These usually come from the (antibiotic- and hormone-containing) meat leftovers that are then processed with sodium, nitrates, and artificial coloring and flavor to make them taste good.

Skip the sliced turkey, salami, ham, roast beef, and other deli meats and eat fresh meat like roast turkey or chicken.

3. Diet/low-fat foods: A perfect example of good food gone bad, many of these foods actually often have more sugar, salt, and unhealthy fillers so they don't taste like something from which all the flavor has been removed. Then people double down on their serving size because they think the food is healthy or because it isn't as satisfying as the real thing. One homemade chocolate chip cookie is going to make a sweet tooth happier than a dozen of the so-called fat free (read high-sugar) variety.

4. By-products or foods left over from corn processing and repurposed into edibles: Corn is sometimes referred to as "yellow gold" because it is used to make so many products and by-products that end up everywhere from food store shelves to gas pumps to industrial chemical plants. Yum. Corn-based cereals, snack foods, salad dressings, soft drink sweeteners, chewing gum, and peanut butter made with corn, syrup or sugar or corn oil, grits, hominy grits, taco shells, specialty corn, including white corn, blue corn, and popcorn are all pretty much zero for zero when it comes to vitamins and minerals.

Skip the grits and opt for oats, preferably rolled or steel-cut. Make your own popcorn and eliminate anything with corn by-products from your diet.

5. Margarine: Not a healthy alternative to butter, this vegetable oil product is weighed down with trans fats, which increase cholesterol.

Skip the spread and eat olive oil or, in small amounts, butter instead.

6. Fast-food chains: The very things that make it fast and cheap are what make this kind of meal unhealthy. It's generally loaded with sodium and artificial sweeteners and preservatives.

Skip the mass produced and eat real food. This doesn't mean you have to cook a full course meal. There are local fast food restaurants, or buy a low-sodium roasted chicken or turkey at the supermarket.

7. Frozen packaged meals: They may be more convenient than sliced bread, but they are usually highly processed and overflowing with fat and salt.

Skip the packaged meals in the freezer section and head over to the frozen veggies instead (look for those without added salt and sauces). Cook up a batch of grains and freeze. Mix and match to make salads, soups, omelets, and casseroles throughout the week.

8. Soda: This drink is sugar with a bubble problem. Devoid of any nutritional value, it's a leading cause of obesity and diabetes. The sugar-free variety is no better and has been found to lead to packing on pounds as drinkers think their diet soda habit gives them free license to overeat other high-sugar snacks.

Skip all sodas and whip up a nutritious green smoothie instead. Or just drink water.

9. Soy protein isolate: This hyperrefined, nutrient-stripped soy product actually acts a lot like a dose of estrogen on the body and may increase the risk of cancers and infertility in women and is best avoided.

Skip the soy "meats" such as tofurkey and soy milk and eat natural sources of soy like edamame, tofu, and tempeh.

The No-Cleanse Smoothie Regimen

Changing the way you think—and eat—doesn't happen overnight, or in three, five, fourteen, or however many days you decide to cleanse. This is why sticking to a healthy eating plan between cleanses is actually more important than cleansing itself. These green smoothie strategies will get you eating healthfully and nutritiously 24/7, no cleanse or diet required.

There's nothing wrong with eating between meals as long as it's smart snacking. Instead of mindlessly reaching for your favorite junk food, whipping up a green smoothie when hunger hits is a better way to stay on a healthy-eating track.

Green smoothies also make a much better nightcap than alcohol or hot milk because they are filling and easy to digest, so you'll stay satisfied without the heavy, full feeling (and guilt) late-night snacking gives.

Mom was right—breakfast is the most important meal of the day. Not being a morning eater is no excuse not to start your day on the right note. A green smoothie made with a dollop of protein (see page 67) will get your morning mojo moving and keep you energized for hours.

Adding one different superfood to your smoothie every time will give your diet a daily nutrition boost while keeping your green smoothie drinking habit from slipping into a rut. Just about any brightly colored vegetable or fruit qualifies, but there are 21 superfoods in particular—certainly enough to keep your green smoothies from slipping into a bland routine—that are rich in essential fatty acids (EFAs), antioxidants, and/or fiber:

- Alliums such as onions, garlic, and leeks
- Apples
- Avocados
- Beets
- Berries: acai berries, blueberries, raspberries
- Cruciferous vegetables: cabbages, cauliflower, broccoli rabe
- Dark chocolate
- Figs
- Flaxseed
- Ginger
- Green tea
- Horseradish
- Miso
- Red bell peppers
- Seaweed: hijiki, wakame, kelp, nori
- Sesame seeds
- Spices and herbs like turmeric, oregano, thyme, and cinnamon
- Sweet potatoes
- Walnuts
- Whole grains
- Yogurt

Less is more with all smoothie add-ins, even superfoods. You want your green smoothies to stay within three digits when it comes to calorie count. One pound equals around 3,500 calories, which is how many calories you need to cut in order to lose a pound. To put that into perspective, a classic 16-ounce glass of fresh green smoothie made just with water and the 60:40 fruit to green leafy vegetable ratio is 300 calories (depending on what kind of fruit you use), around ½ cup of walnuts equals about 350 calories, and 1 cup of plain nonfat yogurt weighs in at around 135 calories.

PART III

GETTING CLEANSED

· ·

CHAPTER TWELVE

One-Day Reboot Cleanse

This is the antidote for when you have a special event to attend this weekend and your outfit's a tad bit snug; you look and feel as perky as a three-day old cup of coffee; you have been non-stop on the go before, during, and after hours; the last green thing you put in your mouth was a stick of apple-flavored gum; you have the grandmother of all hangovers; you haven't worked out in so long that your sneakers have cobwebs; you're more run down than a cell phone with one bar; you're tired of waking up feeling fat, bloated, and mad at yourself for overdoing it. Take that, vending machine!

A mere 24 hours' worth of cleansing does not exactly seem like it could possibly be enough to have any lasting effect, let alone address any of the above. But bad behavior happens to good people, and a one-day stint is just the (meal) plan to reset and kick in long-term shifts in how you live your life. Our bodies are naturally designed to heal themselves and regenerate. So this cleanse isn't a cure-all; instead, think of it's a fresh start, a mini break from your usual revel of caffeine, booze, processed foods, gluten, sugar, or whatever irritant you feel may be plaguing your body. By telling you what to drink and when to drink it, the cleanse is designed to give you the motivational tools to feel back in control, which, in turn, can help you to break unhealthy habits and start new positive ones. It's short and simple, so most people are able to find time in their schedule and stick to it, whether they are novice or experienced cleansers.

The mono food plan is at the core of the One-Day Reboot Cleanse success. Basically, you use one type of raw leafy vegetable and one type of fruit in your green smoothie for the whole day. The idea is to give you and your body a break from whatever you have been shoving in to it. If you have made it this far into this book, then it should hopefully be obvious that you cannot and should not look for sustenance on a mono diet for more than one day as it won't serve up the full buffet of protein, vitamins, minerals, and all of the other nutrients your body needs to function.

The Practicals

Best Green Smoothie Choices: None. For the One-Day Reboot Cleanse, stick with the Classic Green Smoothie (see Recipe Box, page 221).

- The ideal daily quantity of green smoothie is four glasses (1 quart) for the day. If this is too much, drink what you can.
- In addition to the 32 ounces of Classic Green Smoothie, make sure you drink around 2 quarts of water throughout the day (room temperature will be easier to get down than ice cold). You can spritz it up with some extra ingredients (see Water Flavorings, page 132) or warm it up and add a wedge of lemon or a tablespoon of lemon juice if you're craving a hot drink. (You could drink seltzer, but do you really need to add to your evacuations?)
- Aim to drink every two to three hours, alternating between smoothies and water.

- Try to choose a day when you're able to take it easy and relax, nap, and de-stress. Think of it as a be-kind-to-yourself day.

The Skinny on the Plan

KISS: Keep It Simple, Sweetie. One day, one type of raw leafy vegetable, one type of fruit. That's it. Think: the power of one.

- Kick off the morning with a mug of hot water and lemon.
- A couple of hours later, make your first smoothie (you can make the entire batch for the day and refrigerate).
- Continue alternating between smoothie and water every two to three hours for the remainder of the day.
- Finish with another hot water and lemon as a nightcap.

Cheat Move: Begin your fast in the evening, right after your last meal. By the time you wake up, half the fast will already be over.

Shopping List

- ❏ 6 cups (1 pound) leafy green vegetables
- ❏ 3 pieces ripe fruit
- ❏ 1 cup fruit and/or vegetables and/or ¼ of herbs per 1 pint of water (optional; see Water Flavorings, page 132)
- ❏ Ice (optional)

Prep Menu

You can jump into the One-Day Reboot cold, as this kind of quickie cleanse is often a panic reaction to what went into your body the day before. You won't lose brownie—or greenie—points, and the cleanse will still have a purifying effect. But if you really want to commit to a regular day of cleansing on a weekly or monthly basis, or whatever fits your calendar, then try to start including at least one-half day of prep. The more time you spend on prepping, the more benefits you'll feel from the cleanse.

The main focus of a one-day cleanse prep is your liver, aka Detox Central. Virtually everything you consume passes through the liver. So the ingredients suggested to prepare for a One-Day Reboot Cleanse lean toward giving this often-overworked organ a little extra help.

INCLUDE THESE FOODS

- Hot water with just-squeezed lemon juice. This will give you a megadose of antioxidants such as vitamin C that help boost liver function.

- At least 60 grams of protein that is omega-3-rich and/or low in saturated fat, such as chicken without the skin, egg whites, fatty fish such as sardines and salmon, and vegetarian sources like beans, nuts, and seeds. The amino acids found in protein are crucial for the liver to be able to remove toxins most efficiently.

- Load up on the kind of fiber found in gluten-free grains such as brown rice and millet and green cruciferous veggies like Brussels sprouts, broccoli, and cabbage. Dark leafy greens are easy for the liver to process and ensure regularity in the bowel department. These ingredients will be the foundation of your green smoothie, so generously introducing them now will make the transition to your cleanse easier physically and mentally.

- Nuts like almonds and pecans make a great snack pre-cleanse as they will pump your body with B vitamins such as thiamine, which helps your body withstand stress.

- Legumes such as lentils make a good main meal meat substitute and also come with a high supply of those stress-busting B vitamins.

EXCLUDE THESE FOODS

- Caffeine.
- Fatty proteins like red meat, egg yolks, ground turkey, seafood, and dairy products.
- Alcohol.
- Cigarettes.
- Sugar.
- Wheat products, which can be a common allergen and slow down the liver.
- Fruit. You will be getting more than enough fruit over the next 24 hours, and while fruit is definitely on the USDA's "Must Eat More" list, it is also high in sugars, so a little moderation pre-cleanse is not a bad thing

PERFECT PRE-CLEANSE MENU PLAN

Breakfast: Egg white omelet with chopped spinach or kale.

Lunch: Sardines and dark green salad (no dressing).

Dinner: Roast chicken breast with skin removed, lentils sautéed with dark leafy greens and pecans and mixed with brown rice.

Snacks: Nuts, 1 avocado, roasted chickpeas (very lightly coat with olive oil and a splash of salt and any favorite herb or spice, and roast on a baking sheet in a 400°F oven for 20 minutes until crunchy), kale chips (toss torn de-stemmed kale leaves with a teaspoon of olive oil and 1 minced garlic clove; broil for about 1 minute until crisp).

One-Day Reboot Sample Menu

Mix things up to your Iron Chef's heart's content using the Master Green Smoothie template in the Recipe Box (page 221) or your own favorite mono green smoothie recipe, but this tried-and-true plan will help keep you on a clean track.

Wake-Up Call: A drink of hot water with a splash of lemon juice

Breakfast: Using the Master Green Smoothie proportions in the Recipe Box, blend kale, frozen pineapple, one half coconut milk and one half water, ginger and honey OR spinach, banana, water, unsweetened chocolate, and agave syrup

Make It to Lunch Snack: A drink of hot water with a splash of lemon juice

Lunch: The same smoothie you made for breakfast

Mid-Day Slump Snack: A drink of hot water with a splash of lemon juice or flavored water (see Water Flavorings, page 132)

Dinner: The same smoothie you made for breakfast and lunch

Night-Time Munchies Snack: A drink of hot water with a splash of lemon juice or the same flavored water you had mid-day

Post-Cleanse Clean-Up Menu

Follow the Perfect Prep-Cleanse Menu Plan. The essence of the One-Day Reboot is simplicity. Think of it as your no-brainer plan to better eating.

Quick Tips

These tips will make your One-Day Reboot Cleanse a piece of cake.

SIMPLE STRESS SOLUTIONS

- When you reset on a one-day cleanse, you're not just giving your body a break from the daily grind of eating, you're also giving your mind a day off. Here's how to stop the mental madness:

- Tone down the tunes. Muzak and classical music have been proven to have soothing effects (the latter can be equivalent to taking 10mg of valium).

- Practice breathing. Deep breaths in through the nose and out through the mouth have been shown to relax both the body and mind. Alternatively, take one long breath in through the mouth and exhale in three short bursts through the nose for more mindful breathing to help re-energize.

- Unplug and turn off. Your media may keep you in touch 24/7, but it also interferes with everything from how well you sleep to how well you play with others. Logging off for the time that you're doing a One-Day Reboot Cleanse can be enough to deactivate your mind.

- Sensitize yourself. Add a few drops of rosemary oil and lavender essential oils to a hanky or small cloth and take sniffs throughout the day. Both of these ingredients have been found to calm nerves and help chase away tension.

- Aim to get eight hours of sleep a night.

- Try not to drink after 7 p.m.

- Try this old wives' remedy: Take a warm bath with two cups of Epsom salt dissolved in the water. The salt's key component, magnesium, supports hundreds of enzymes (translation: the stuff that makes our bodies work) in the body.

WATCH OUT FOR

- Boredom. This will probably be your biggest threat. Just keep reminding yourself that this is less than 24 hours of your life.

- Discouragement. No cleanse should have to live up to the results you would get from being on a diet, but the One-Day Reboot Cleanse is the smallest loser of the group when it comes to taking off the pounds. Be realistic—it lasts less than a day. So you will most likely weigh in at a pound or two lighter.

- You'll feel like you're drinking a salad for breakfast (as well as lunch and dinner, but the first meal of the day seems to be the most difficult when it comes to drinking your greens).

- You may feel a little light-headed.

PAYOFF

- You reboot your body, which helps you to feel lighter and brighter, like a more healthy and energized you. Ideally, these buoyant feelings will overflow into the other six days of your week and get you into a healthy frame of mind.

- Although the initial weight loss is on the light side and has the potential to pile back on, a One-Day Reboot Cleanse is a smooth gateway to eating a healthier, more balanced diet in general.

- This is actually the easiest of the cleanses whether you're wet behind the ears or you're an old hand when it comes to smoothie cleanses. Many people make it a weekly ritual.

- It may be difficult the first time, but if you make the One-Day Reboot Cleanse a weekly ritual, it really is one of those things that gets easier with practice (as opposed to calculus).

- You're giving your body a much-needed one-day break from the usual demands that you place on it.
- By the mid-afternoon smoothie, you'll be surprisingly full and struggling to drink every drop.
- A one-day cleanse is an extremely efficient way to reboot. You don't have to slowly work your way in or out of it like you do with the longer cleanses. It will last just long enough before the cleansing process starts to get really serious.
- Even a quickie one-day cleanse is enough to make you feel in control and short circuit bad habits.

CHAPTER THIRTEEN

Three-Day Blast Cleanse

What makes this cleanse especially effective is that it's just short enough that anyone can do it, but still packs a cleansing wallop to get the job done. In just 72 hours, you can drink your way to a healthier body and lifestyle.

Yes, losing weight is a part of this cleanse—often as much as 5 pounds. But it isn't actually the point of the cleanse. Not everyone needs to lose weight; everyone needs to feel better. Seriously. Feeling sluggish about your weight isn't really about piling on the pounds. The true root of the problem is having low energy because of your diet. We eat for all sorts of reasons, and very rarely because we are actually hungry. Sometimes we reach for food to soothe our emotional cravings. When we are anxious, angry, fatigued, overwhelmed, or otherwise under stress, a hard-to-resist desire to overeat can take over.

Unfortunately, the foods we crave tend to be the quick fixes: sugary, salty, fatty, or full of carbs. They don't provide any fuel, so your body feels heavy and draggy, which causes you to move less but keep on eating the same amount, making it more difficult to get up and go, which causes your body to feel even heavier and draggier, and so on.

The Three-Day Blast reverses this downward spiral and motivates you to take care of yourself.

The idea is that over the course of the three days, you become connected with your body in a way that makes you hyperaware of when you feed it, what you feed it, why you're feeding it at that moment, and how it feels after you have fed it. Instead of your pre-cleanse tendency of serving yourself huge portions and eating without thinking (I have always had coffee with cream and sugar so why would I stop having coffee with cream and sugar?), you become conscious of every morsel of food that passes your lips. After the cleanse, you feel less compelled to overindulge and, when you do reach for something to eat, you're more likely to nourish yourself with a greener, cleaner diet of water, whole vegetables, whole fruits, and leaner proteins. Since you're not trying to live on a diet of heavy foods full of highly processed ingredients, white sugars, carbs, salt, fats, and/or food with minimal nutritional value, you naturally will have more energy and vitality.

The best part of this mini cleanse? There's no calorie counting or dieting involved. Nor do you have limit yourself to drinking the same smoothie three times a day for three days. However, some types of green smoothies are more nourishing than others and therefore better suited for energizing you for the duration of the cleanse, so try to follow the general recipe suggestions.

The Practicals

Best Green Smoothie Choices: You'll want to choose smoothies that are high in protein for breakfast—look for recipes marked as "high-protein"; a good range of flavors will get you through the afternoon slump, such as anything with tropical fruit or lots of add-ins; go for a slightly thicker combo for dinner, such as smoothies that incorporate grains, nuts, and seeds; and opt for a sweet end to the day—look for smoothies in the desserts portion of the Recipe Box (page 221).

- Each green smoothie "meal" should be 12 to 16 ounces. If this is too much to drink in one sitting (surprisingly, it can be), then spread it out throughout the day.

- Drink at least 16 ounces of water after each "meal." Make sure you're drinking plenty of water throughout the day (aim for a minimum of 2 quarts). Add fresh lemon juice to give it a zesty flavor or drink it hot, if you prefer.

- The best time to fit a three-day cleanse into an average work schedule is to begin Friday morning and continue through to Sunday night. This way you can take it easy for the last day, which tends to be the hardest, break the cleanse with a light dinner Sunday evening, and be bright-eyed and bushy-tailed for work Monday morning.

- Try to finish the last smoothie at least three hours before bedtime.

- Plan on getting your heart pumping. Gently. You may be feeling light-headed, so your usual workout routine could leave you feeling nauseous and dizzy. But try to go for a walk or relax with some very gentle yoga poses. For no-sweat ways to get your circulation going, turn your shower into a Scandanavian shower experience by switching between hot and cold water and scrubbing your skin with a shower salt or loofah.

Cheat Move: If your aim is to lose weight, skip the nut milks, juices, and other liquids and stick with water as your green smoothie fluid base. You won't miss the added flavor because the green smoothies are pretty tasty with just leafy vegetables and fruit. If you want a thicker consistency, just have it on the (crushed) rocks.

Shopping List

- ❑ 3 to 5 pounds leafy green vegetables
- ❑ 2 pounds other vegetables
- ❑ 9 pieces of ripe fruit: 3 should be on the sweeter side such as mangoes, bananas, cherries, figs, or tangerines
- ❑ Water Flavorings (page 132) for up to six 8-ounce cups
- ❑ Small chunk gingerroot (about 2 inches)
- ❑ 2 lemons
- ❑ 1 to 2 cups protein (see page 67 for suggestions)
- ❑ 6 tablespoons sweetener (honey, Stevia, or agave nectar)
- ❑ Ice (optional)

Shopping Tip: Good starter produce for any Three-Day Blast Cleanse green smoothie—spinach, red pepper, carrots, bananas, avocado, pineapple, cucumber, cauliflower, pumpkin puree.

Prep Menu

You'll need to blast off with a diet makeover at least a day and a half before you start the actual cleanse. The reality is that you will be actually green smoothie-ing for a short period of time. (Sure, it may not feel so speedy while you're actually doing it, but time is relative—especially when you are measuring it by the glassful of blended veggies and fruit). So easing into your stripped-down diet will not only make the next 72 hours much easier, it will also make your efforts more likely to succeed.

Your key word is "elimination." The idea is to limit or completely lose your intake of processed sugars, refined carbohydrates, full-fat dairy foods like cheese and ice cream, artificial sweeteners, gluten (mainly white foods such as rice and bread), saturated fats such as red meat, caffeine, and alcohol. The simplest guideline is: If it's something a college student would eat for breakfast, then it's something you probably shouldn't be eating any time leading up to your cleanse. The easiest way to stop the culinary madness is to start gradually reducing the amounts of sugar, salt, fat, and starch you take in for a week or so before you begin your cleanse, strategizing so that you are on a sin-free diet 36 hours before you whip up your first green smoothie. At the same time, increase your water intake. This slo-mo switch-and-bait approach will stop you from feeling like you are going into withdrawals during the cleanse.

The Skinny on the Plan

This cleanse is all about refreshment. Seriously. You are revitalizing your body and mind by revamping your diet. This means that the menu you follow while on a Three-Day Blast Cleanse should be made from ingredients that stay away from the four deadly eating sins: foods that are sugary, starchy (carbs), suety (fat), and salty.

- The day before you start the cleanse, grate the ginger to make ½ cup. Then quarter two of the lemons, remove the seeds and mix with ginger and the sweetener. Steep in 48 ounces of boiled water at least 1 hour. Strain and store in the refrigerator.
- Upon rising, wake up your brain and your taste buds with a mug of heated up ginger-lemon tea.
- Breakfast is still the most important meal of the day, so power up with a Super Protein Green Smoothie.
- Drink water throughout the day (see Water Flavorings, page 132, for ideas).
- At lunchtime, drink up a full-flavored green smoothie packed with lots of complex flavors.
- For a midday snack, drink another lemon-ginger tea.
- Don't stop drinking water.
- For dinner, relax with a chunkier smoothie choice that will keep you full.
- Finish off with a sweet dessert green smoothie.
- Repeat for the next two days, but vary the green smoothie recipes if you want.

INCLUDE THESE FOODS

Lots of strong flavors as you eliminate. This will stop your taste buds from staging a late-night munchies rebellion. Instead of drinking plain water, flavor it with lemon or lime juice, ginger, or cucumber; eat sweet potato instead of plain potato, beets instead of carrots, kale instead of lettuce, brown rice instead of oats, fish and lean white meat seasoned with turmeric, curry, cayenne, or any spice that makes your tongue tingle.

EXCLUDE THESE FOODS

Those four "S" food groups: Salty, sweet, suety, and starchy foods—your daily total should be less than 1,200 grams of sodium, less than 20 grams of sugar, less than 40 grams of fat, and less than 200 grams of carbs.

PERFECT 36-HOUR PRE-CLEANSE MENU PLAN

Sprinkle some of these ingredients on every meal: spices and flavorings like nutmeg, cinnamon, allspice, cayenne, turmeric, rosemary, curry, lavender, hot pepper, pepper, garlic, mint, vanilla, lemon and/or lime juice, paprika, lemon balm, lemongrass, or whatever adds zip to your day.

Day 1

Breakfast: Try to make it at least 50 percent fruit or vegetable such as fresh berries with low-fat yogurt, avocado on a brown rice cracker, or brown rice and mango.

Morning Snack: Flavored water or green tea steeped with herb sprigs, plus 1 cup of berries.

Lunch: Salad with fruit, greens, chickpeas, and nuts, no dressing, plus 1 cup of grains.

Midafternoon Snack: Flavored water and hummus with veggies.

Dinner: Raw or steamed broccoli sprinkled with sunflower or pumpkin seeds, cooked grains flavored with nut or avocado oil, or lentils, and a piece of fruit.

Bedtime Snack: Green tea flavored with herb sprigs and 10 almonds.

Day 2

Breakfast: Egg white vegetable omelet and glass of pulpy orange juice.

Morning Snack: 1 cup of berries.

Lunch: Wrap brown rice and chopped veggies in lettuce.

Three-Day Blast Sample Menu

Follow your taste buds into the Recipe Box (page 221) or use your own trip-the-flavor-fandango green smoothie recipes, but this guideline will keep your three-day cleanse balanced with just the right amount of sweet and spicy.

Wake-Up Call: A drink of sweetened hot water flavored with lemon juice and steeped with ginger.

Breakfast: Choose one of following each day: Protein-Fiber Morning Power Punch (page 226), Vermont Stack (page 227), or the No Time for Breakfast Smoothie (page 227).

Make It to Lunch Snack: A drink of flavored water.

Lunch: Choose one of following each day: Ranch House Salad (page 227), Green Chai Latte (page 232), or "I Hate Vegetables" (page 237).

Mid-Day Slump Snack: A drink of hot water with a splash of lemon juice or flavored water (see Water Flavorings, page 132).

Dinner: Choose one of following each day: Masala Curry (page 231), Chinese Take-Out (page 230), or Nachos Bar Food (page 229).

Night-Time Munchies Snack: Choose one of following each day: Thanksgiving Pumpkin Pie (page 235), Berry Berry Pie (page 236), or Cosmopolitan Cocktail (page 239).

Post-Cleanse Clean-Up Menu

Add the following to your smoothie menu. Eat for at least one and a half days, but ideally two to three days:

Day 1: A few pieces of fruit, raw or lightly steamed vegetables, leafy green salad, 1 cup of cooked grains such as quinoa or brown rice.

Day 2 : Follow Day 1 and add a bowl of yogurt or kefir.

Day 3: Follow Day 2 and add a maximum of two poached or boiled eggs, 4 ounces of either poached or baked white fish or roasted chicken.

QUICK TIPS

These tips will make your Three-Day Blast Cleanse pass in a flash:

You will have cravings. What is important to remember is that you never feel better after succumbing. But understanding why you want (fill in your go-to junk food) right this moment will help you withstand them. Cravings can have different triggers depending on the time of the day:

- Morning: You may not have eaten enough to sustain you at breakfast. Fight it by having another protein-powered smoothie.

- Mid-morning: This is usually a reaction to caffeine withdrawal. Stave it off with a ginger-lemon tea.

- Afternoon: As the day's stresses catch up, the body starts to cry out for its edible comfy blanket—carbs or sweets. If you can't mentally muscle through, eat a pear, banana, or some grapes, all of which will satisfy both cravings.

- Evening: It's de-stress time! Unfortunately, we often turn to snack foods and/or booze to help us relax. Add some filling grains to your night-time dessert smoothie and add a twist of fruit to give it a "Sex on the Beach" flair.

Don't make life hard(er) on yourself. Check your calendar before planning your cleanse to make sure that you don't have any special events that weekend.

Along the same lines, don't end up in a place where getting to the toilet can be a challenge, like an airplane or a drive out in the country. You will need (plenty) of easy access.

Cleanse when:

- You feel like a slug has more energy than you.
- You find yourself aimlessly eating all the time, even when you're not hungry, and you want to reevaluate what you're putting into your body.
- You realize that you have gone up a size since last season (a caveat that you will still need to go shopping for a new wardrobe if you revert back to your old eating habits post-cleanse).

A recent study found that people who lose a significant amount of weight early in a diet are most successful in the long-term. It creates confidence and momentum that carries over to sticking to the plan. So to help keep off any pounds that the cleanse quick-blasted off, gradually start eating after the cleanse by replacing one of your daily smoothies with a solid meal the first day, then two green smoothies with solid meals and so on.

WATCH OUT FOR

Killer headaches and hunger pangs. While normal, they can make it hard to focus. If you feel like you're about to bail, go ahead and make an extra green smoothie and see if that helps you stay the course.

The third day of any cleanse tends to be the hardest, which can make it a down day to end your cleanse. From the moment you wake up, you'll probably notice a dip in energy. This is when you're most likely to feel fuzzy-headed, sluggish, and irritable (think a three-year-old in need of a nap). The smoothie schedule is now predictable...and therefore, predictably unexciting. A midday nap can sometimes get you through to the other side.

It's the weekend, but it won't be time for you to get your party on. It's hard enough cleansing for three days without adding the extra challenge of surrounding yourself with friends who have not seen the cleansing light. Who cares that their "drink, eat, and be merry" lifestyle is setting them up for a mess of pain? It's still no fun to sit on the sidelines and watch.

Accept that this will be the weekend that there's birthday cake at work in the morning, afternoon, and at the end of the day, your mom/partner/neighbor will make your favorite fried food for dinner; and the movies have a special free popcorn promotion. Life is full of willpower tests. The take-away from this cleanse isn't Chinese food or that you now have a quick way to drop a few pounds instantly. It's learning that saying yes to healthier foods isn't denying yourself, it's taking care of yourself.

THE PAYOFF

This isn't a diet, so there's no calorie counting. As long as you stay away from commercial smoothies, which are chockablock with unhealthy additives, you can't really overindulge on a green smoothie. Yes, as far as weight gain is concerned, a calorie is a calorie whether it comes from a chocolate bar or a cup of pulverized vegetables and fruit. But there are a heap of reasons to base your food choices on measures other than calorie count. For example, green smoothies wrack up the fiber, which is going to leave you feeling full longer so you'll consume fewer calories overall. In fact, the benefit of making green smoothies a regular part of your diet is that the vegetables and fruit that make up their bulk give you more bang for your buck. Carbohydrates and protein have 4 calories per gram, while fats have more than twice as much: an entire 9 calories per gram. (Alcohol weighs in at 7 calories per gram.) If you're on the calorie-count treadmill to lose weight, but you're eating higher-fat foods like bacon and full-fat cheese, you could potentially consume over half your day's calorie allotment by the end of breakfast. Choosing carbs and protein for your morning meal, on the other hand, like a green smoothie made with leafy greens, blueberries, and some low-fat yogurt, will leave you with calories to spare the entire day.

Repeat: This isn't a diet. But if you continue to create a healthy new lifestyle, you'll probably continue to lose weight even after the cleanse. You'll crave the kinds of food that are good for you and give you long-term satisfaction—like salads, fish, and vegetables—rather than giving in to short-term urges.

You get quick payback as you lose your water bloat within the first day while you still feel great. These are the sort of results you won't want to undo once you're off the cleanse, which is a great motivator for staying with the cleanse for the full three days and continuing to eat well after.

Even when you slip back into your old ways and indulge in a Boston cream donut or a plate of nachos and fake cheese or whatever your food noir is—which you'll most likely do at least once or twice simply because you see it and you have been conditioned for so long to think that this type of eating can satisfy you—you'll quickly regret it. Not just in a guilty "why did I do that" mental beat-yourself-up way, but really and truly physically regret it as your body rejects the sudden influx of toxic artificial flavorings.

CHAPTER FOURTEEN

Five-Day
Fine-Tune Cleanse

OK, it's time to get serious. A Five-Day Fine-Tune Cleanse isn't a Three-Day Blast plus two. This cleanse works by an entirely different playbook. It's only for those who have cleared at least one multiday cleanse or the strong-minded first-time cleansers who are feeling ambitious and want to see major results.

One way this cleanse differs from others is that it isn't about cutting out foods: it's about adding more food and having it more often. You're still operating in a liquefied world, but the longer length of time that you're on the cleanse means that you'll need more—much more—to sustain your body and your mind. The Five-Day Fine-Tune Cleanse is designed to balance your energy by feeding it. It's based on a concept developed by researchers who found that our bodies do better with a constant and steady stream of healthy calories rather than the three times a day pile-on-your-plate-pile-in-your-mouth eating plan most of us tend to follow (plus snacking in between). People with the largest energy imbalances (those whose calorie surpluses or shortfalls topped 500 calories from hour to hour) lean toward being the unhealthiest, while those who keep within an hourly surplus or deficit of 300 to 500 calories at all times are likely to have the most balanced energy levels, more lean muscle mass, and less body fat. This makes sense, as your body is never pushed to the point of panicky, running-on-empty, out-of-control hunger because you're topping it up often with healthy fuel.

In addition to never feeling hungry on this cleanse, this more constant eating plan will lead to a flood of new energy and a reconnection to a more youthful, rested you. Think of it as pressing the reboot button on your eating and drinking habits. So if you want to look slimmer, feel fitter, and live longer, then eat—or, in this case, drink—green smoothies more often.

After you finish your five-day feeding binge, your diet will be readjusted and you won't crave your old three-squares-a-day habit. You may have to continue to fine-tune by whipping up a green smoothie when the urge strikes to put yourself out of the 300 to 500 calorie range. Green smoothies make potent meal substitutes and satisfying healthy snacks, so it will be easy to keep your intake within that recommended range. Once you're post-cleanse, get in the habit of switching out one meal or a couple of snacks a day with one of the green smoothies from the Recipe Box (page 221) and you'll keep your stomach full, which will reduce the likelihood of returning to your old diet of scheduled gorging.

The Practicals

Best Green Smoothie Choices: Diversify, diversify, and diversify. Drink the same green smoothie for every meal and snack or even for every meal time, like breakfast, and even the most delicious blend is going to start to resemble a cup of greens after they have been strained through an old gym sock. You'll be drinking a lot of smoothies over the next 120 hours, so make the Recipe Box (page 221) your favorite reading material (green smoothie recipes marked with 5D mean they make ideal drinks for this cleanse).

- Mixing up your green smoothie flavors throughout the day can be a challenge, especially if you're away from home all day. But staying not just engaged in your cleanse but also enjoying it—as opposed to treating each drink time as an item on your cleanse checklist that must be crossed off—will be even more of a challenge if you don't inject a little variety in your smoothies every day.

- Each green smoothie "meal" should be 12 ounces. If this is too much to drink in one sitting (surprisingly, it can be), then spread it out across two hours. You need to fill up to stay in the game.

- The best time to fit a five-day cleanse into an average work schedule is to begin Sunday night and continue through to Friday early evening. This way you can end on TGIF, which tends to be a tough night to make it through on a green smoothie (although after five days, you'll be surprised at how little you'll feel like a plate of buffalo wings).

- Don't skip your workout. You might not put as much burn into your usual plan of action, but you should definitely keep on moving.

Cheat Move: Day three is the killer, so if you're tempted to cave (on this or any day), do it with the same whole foods that you would have added to your smoothie anyway, like an apple, a carrot, or some sugar snap peas.

Shopping List

Rather than a few set green leafy vegetables and fruit, the Five-Day Fine-Tune Cleanse encourages you to focus on a generous market basket of food types to fulfill your core nutritional needs. Follow these simple guidelines to help your body increase lean muscle mass and avoid storing fat while cleansing (or any time):

Vary your food at every "meal" or snack. The more variety you have in your diet while cleansing will make it easier to stick with it for the full five days. You want to aim to get a balanced combination of protein, carbohydrates, and fat in every smoothie. So load up on a variety of produce. For the five days, you will need a minimum of:

- ❑ 10 pounds of leafy green vegetables
- ❑ 4 pounds of other vegetables
- ❑ 18 pieces of ripe fruit
- ❑ 5 measures of fruit, herbs, or vegetables for water (optional; see Water Flavorings, page 132)
- ❑ 4 cups of protein (see page 67 for suggestions)
- ❑ 1 cup of sweetener (honey, stevia, or agave nectar)
- ❑ Ice (optional)

Blend a bit of protein into each snack. It will go a long way toward making you feel not just full, but also full of energy. (Look for anything marked with "high-protein" in the recipes or check out the protein sides in Chapter Six on page 67).

Include two or three foods from the super list below in each of your three major daily "meals" and at least one of them in each of your three daily snacks. They have been proven to boost muscles, help with shedding extra pounds, strengthen bones, lower blood pressure, fight cancer, improve the immune system, and/or fight heart disease:

- ❑ Raw almonds and other nuts
- ❑ Soybeans, chickpeas, and other legumes
- ❑ 100% peanut butter (no added oil, sodium, or sugar)
- ❑ Olive oil
- ❑ Whole grains like quinoa and oats

- ❑ Protein powder like whey
- ❑ Blueberries, raspberries, and other berries
- ❑ Yogurt (only live will do; if you are buying commercial yogurt, make sure it contains the "Live & Active Cultures" seal, which is a simplified way of saying it has lactic-acid-producing bacteria such as Lactobacillus bulgaricus and Streptococcus thermophilus, which can aid in digestion).

Prep Menu

Serious cleanses require serious prep. Begin at least two-and-a-half days before you plan to cleanse. It may seem like you will be getting enough of a good thing once you get going on your fine-tune, but you will have a greater chance of success if you start developing your taste for green smoothies pre-cleanse. So snacks will be pure green—smoothie, that is. This will also help keep you fuller because your main meals will be on the lighter side.

INCLUDE THESE FOODS	EXCLUDE THESE FOODS
Anything that could be a green smoothie ingredient	Everything your mother and doctor warned you against: booze, tobacco, drugs, salty and oily foods (chips, anyone?), candy and other sweet indulgences, anything processed (think margarine, white enriched flour, most pasta), and fast or instant food
Low-fat proteins like the "other meats" (chicken, pork, turkey) without skins, any fish but especially bottom feeders like sardines, mackerel, anchovies, monkey food (nuts and seeds), and that old-man-in-the-diner favorite, egg-whites	
Flavored water (see Water Flavorings, page 132)	

The Skinny on the Plan

This is the cleanse that proves the naysayers wrong. You will never feel deprived, like you are on a diet or as if you are dying of starvation on the Fine-Tuner. You drink and then you drink and then you drink some more. There is nothing wrong with loading up at the buffet if you keep to foods that are green, lean, and clean—in other words, a diet that is kind to your body.

- Start drinking your first smoothie for breakfast and then have another smoothie approximately every two hours until about two hours before you sink into bed for the night.
- Every other smoothie should have a protein boost to keep your energy levels fighting fit.
- Drink as much hot or cold water as you think you need (see Drink Up and Water Flavorings).

PERFECT 2–TO 3-DAY PRE-CLEANSE MENU PLAN

Choose one from each section for each meal and snack.

Breakfast: Oatmeal and fruit, scrambled egg whites with salsa and veggies, or any smoothie from the Recipe Box (page 221).

Morning Snack: Any smoothie from the Recipe Box or ¼ cup raw nuts.

Lunch: Green salad with lentils and raw vegetables, or carrot ginger soup (or any chopped vegetable soup) sprinkled with raw sunflower seeds and four rice crackers, or mixed bean salad lightly coated with tahini, or any smoothie from the Recipe Box.

Midafternoon Snack: Sliced vegetables dipped in tahini, black beans pureed with garlic, or tomato salsa

Dinner: Curried lentils with brown rice and raw cashews, or small piece of salmon with grains and steamed vegetables, or any smoothie from the Recipe Box.

Bedtime Snack: Any smoothie from the Recipe Box or pureed frozen fruit

Five-Day Fine-Tune Sample Menu

This is green smoothies, all day, all the time, so mix things up to keep your tummy full and your body healthy. Drink flavored water (see Water Flavorings, page 132) throughout the day as needed.

Wake-Up Call: A drink of sweetened hot water flavored with lemon juice and steeped with ginger.

Breakfast: Choose one of following each day: More-Than-Grapefruit (page 225), Almost Cup of Joe (page 226), Goldilocks Smoothie (page 226), Ginger, Oat, and Berry Breakfast (page 238), or Very Berry (page 231).

Make It to Lunch Snack: Choose one of following each day: Protein-Fiber Morning Power Punch (page 226), Peanut Butter and Jelly (page 232), Pre-Workout (page 236), or the No Time for Breakfast Smoothie (page 227).

Lunch: Choose any variation each day from the Master Green Smoothie (page 223).

Midday Slump Snack: Choose one of following each day: Post-Workout (page 236), Stop the Clog (if needed; page 237), Stop the Trots (if needed; page 237), Sometimes You Feel Like a Nut (page 238), Fruity Multivitamin Dinner (page 239).

Dinner: Choose any variation each day from the Master Green Smoothie list (page 223).

Night-Time Munchies Snack: Happy Hour Smoothie (page 233).

Post-Cleanse Clean-Up Menu

Eat for at least two-and-a-half days, but ideally three to five days

Days 1–3: Eat only vegetables, fruits, nuts, seeds, lentils, plant-based oils, and seasonings.

Day 4: Introduce white fish, legumes, beans and grains such as brown rice, quinoa, and oats; go easy on the salt.

Day 5: Add eggs and or soy (such as tofu or edamame) to your menu.

Quick Tips

Green and white tea (unroasted green tea) with lemon slices won't only detox you, they can help you sail through the five stages of coffee withdrawal that your body goes through over the course of five days:

Day 1: Crankiness

Day 2: Headaches, headaches, headaches

Day 3: Fatigue

Day 4: Total lack of concentration

Day 5: Crankiness, headaches, fatigue, trouble concentrating

Otherwise, herbal teas without caffeine, such as dandelion root tea, or Alka-Tea, which contains 49 alkalinizing wild-crafted herbs, are energizing choices.

Greens smoothies tend to satisfy a sweet tooth, so after a few days you're more likely to start fantasizing about Saltines, pretzels, potato chips, and other salty snacks. You could lick your arm after working up a sweat, but much less strange is to satisfy your sodium urges by free-styling some seaweed in your green smoothie.

WATCH OUT FOR

Poop. Lots and lots of poop. However much you think you will expel, multiply as it will be so much more. Plus lots and lots of pee. Translation: Stick close to the toilet or invest in a bulk pack of adult diapers.

The Monday effect. There's actually a scientific reason for the Monday morning blues. Our internal clocks naturally tick on a day that is longer than 24 hours. By the time Monday winds around each week, we've built up a sleep deficit of at least an hour. So before starting your five-day cleanse, fine-tune your sleep time by scheduling to hit the sack an hour earlier Sunday night or staying horizontal an hour longer Monday morning.

Organizational stress. The need for smoothie variety means you'll need to think and plan your drinks ahead. You may end up having to pack as many as four to six smoothies to carry with you if you're away from home most of the day.

THE PAYOFF

Five days means you'll have more time to realign. Three days aren't always helpful to making dietary changes.

Once you work through the Monday start, this cleanse dovetails nicely with most people's work schedules; you will be occupied during most of the cleanse, which will make the time practically speed by (not really, but it will pass more quickly).

You'll crave Brussels sprouts (or something similar) during and afer the cleanse.

You'll eat healthier after the cleanse because you now know you can.

Five days of green smoothies can point out just how out of whack your everyday diet might be: too much bland starch, too much heavy meat, too much processed sugar, too much caffeine, too much alcohol, and nowhere near enough fresh produce.

CHAPTER FIFTEEN

Two-Week
Full-Body Cleanse

First of all, here's who this cleanse isn't for: someone who has not cleansed before. Sure, you're hardcore and more goal-oriented than a 14-year-old boy playing "Angry Birds" on his iPad. But if you have not tried a green smoothie cleanse before, this isn't the way to start. At the very least you're setting up yourself up for a tough time and possibly failure because you don't really understand what you're signing up for. There's a lot to be said for the slow and steady approach.

However, if you have happily swum in the green smoothie swamp waters and want to dip your toes in deeper, this is a an ideal cleanse for rebalancing your life and your diet. Think of it as hitting your three R's: Renew. Revitalize. Rebalance.

This kind of cleansing makeover will take a little more commitment than a five-day cleanse, and not just in the number of days. There's much work to be done beyond pulverizing produce. You're doing something good for your mind and soul as well as your body. This is an important point as it's what will get you over the Day 3 slump with a joyful mental leap.

Although there's no scientific basis to the belief that it takes 21 days to form a new habit, two weeks is certainly enough time to establish a comfort level with a new behavior. So taking on the Full-Body Cleanse could be just the jump-start your body and mind need to get back into healthy living. The cleanse includes 14 meaningful yet manageable steps for you to take toward a cleaner state of being. Make one of these changes every day, and when the cleanse is finished, you'll feel like a whole new you. While the Full-Body Cleanse isn't as severe as the Master Cleanse and nowhere near as pricey as a juice fast, don't delude yourself—it does involve more liquid meals than anyone who does not live in Hollywood or has had jaw surgery may have previously experienced. However, because you will be ingesting a similar amount of calories than if you were eating, this is simply a liquid versus solid issue. You won't be hungry. At first, you may crave sweet food. Then salty food. But after a while, it becomes any food…like maybe a salad. Or a bowl of quinoa. Or a beet. A nice, earthy red beet. Yeah, you could really bite into a nice, earthy red beet right now. Get it? You'll crave healthy.

The Practicals

Best Green Smoothie Choices: You'll want to keep to a familiar dietary routine, so think breakfast, snack, lunch, snack, dinner, dessert, and look for green smoothies that will give you those meals' flavor sensations.

- Anticipate that you'll be drinking around 12 glasses of water daily (between smoothies, not during). "Season" as needed (see Water Flavorings, page 132).
- Although you can drink as much green smoothie as you want daily, you probably won't manage more than 1 quart.
- Try to add one probiotic (such as yogurt, miso paste, kefir, microalgae like spirulina, chlorella, and blue-green algae, dark chocolate, and/or tempeh) daily to one of your green smoothies to help keep the natural flora and fauna in your digestive system flourishing over the next two weeks.

The Skinny on the Plan

This is hardcore cleansing, which means you will need to put on your party-planning hat and do everything possible to ensure that your diet pre-, during, and post-cleanse is varied enough to keep you coming back for more.

- Start with two 8-ounce glasses of water when you first wake up, adding a couple of tablespoons of protein powder if you need an extra boost of energy.
- Substitute coconut water for one of your waters after working out.
- Alternate with 12-ounce green smoothies throughout the day.
- Substitute an iced or hot green or herbal tea for a water midday when energy reserves are low.
- The amount of smoothies you drink depends on what you put in them. This cleanse is about drinking to stave off hunger and keep your energy high, not starving yourself.
- Stop all drinking—smoothies and water—two hours before bedtime or you'll be up all night emptying your bladder.

- Make the effort to break a sweat once a day. It will make you feel better. Really.
- Coconut water is a healthy, refreshing sports drink for replenishing electrolytes without added sugar. Not to mention coconut water is packed with vitamin C.
- You have to be very organized and make and bring enough green smoothies with you wherever you go. That means having a way to carry up to a quart of liquid plus keep it cool (see Smoothie Sailing, page 201, for what happens when a green smoothie gets too hot; warning—it ain't pretty).

Cheat Move #1: The water isn't exactly going make your taste buds trip the light fandango, but its important to keep hydrated to feel satiated, flush the waste products your body churns out when processing protein or breaking down fat and transporting nutrients to your muscles, and to keep your metabolism ticking. But if you feel you just can't take another sip, switch to green or herbal tea (made from ginger, lemon, and/or herbs like mint, parsley, and lemon balm).

Cheat Move #2: If you fold before the 14 days are up, reset. Greensters would say that technically you should start again from day one. But if you don't consider yourself a Greenster, simply begin the cleanse again from whichever day you stopped. However, you get only one second chance…unless your cheat food was something that is on the green smoothie recipe list. In that case, it doesn't count as a fail and you can continue with your originally scheduled cleanse.

Shopping List

- ❏ Green tea
- ❏ Ice (optional)
- ❏ 14 cups of fruit and/or vegetables and 1½ cups herbs for water (optional; see Water Flavorings, page 132)
- ❏ Big piece of gingerroot
- ❏ 3 cups of whey protein powder
- ❏ 3 liters of coconut water
- ❏ 30 pounds of leafy green vegetables
- ❏ 12 pounds of other vegetables
- ❏ 54 pieces of ripe fruit
- ❏ 12 cups of protein (see page 67 for suggestions)
- ❏ 3 cups of sweetener (honey, stevia, or agave nectar)
- ❏ 14 probiotic foods (yogurt, kefir, microalgae like spirulina, chlorella, and blue-green algae, miso paste, dark chocolate, tempeh, and/or kombucha tea)

Prep Menu

You'll need to factor in at least one prep week pre-cleanse and a one recovery week post-cleanse. In other words, you will be devoting almost a full calendar month to do a two-week cleanse. Which seems like a lot until you take into account that the payback is completely overhauling what you have put in your mouth on a daily basis for the past many years and the outcome will probably add quality years to your life while giving your skin an amazing glow. Then it doesn't seem like quite so much.

INCLUDE THESE FOODS

- Flavored water—you will be surprised at how delicious a cup of H20 spiked with a splash of mint will seem by day 3.
- Lots of low fat protein to keep your energy levels strong—take the skin off of poultry (but skip the commercial roast turkey and all luncheon meats altogether as they tends to be plumped with sodium, nitrates, and sometimes saturated fats), egg whites, low fat yogurt, and omega-rich fish.
- The last thing you want during a four-week menu makeover is to feel clogged—a steady intake of fiber will keep your pipes squeaky clean. Stick with grains such as brown rice and millet, beans such as black and kidney, lentils, fruit like pears and apples, and green cruciferous veggies like Brussels sprouts, broccoli, and cabbage.

EXCLUDE THESE FOODS

- The usual suspects of tobacco, alcohol, and processed foods. The best way to figure out if an ingredient doesn't belong in your cleanse? If it has more than one ingredient, if it requires processing to make it edible, or if it was not eaten in pre-Industrial times, take it off the menu.

PERFECT TWO-WEEK PRE-CLEANSE MENU PLAN

Breakfast Ideas: Switch your normal cup of coffee for a mug of green tea, a bowl of hot whole grains like quinoa or barley, or some steel-cut oatmeal jazzed up with honey or maple syrup and cinnamon, or a poached egg on top of steamed asparagus.

Morning, Afternoon, and Evening Snack Ideas: You can choose any of the below suggestions when snack time comes around.

- 10 to 15 raw almonds
- Apple or pear, sliced, with 1 tablespoon raw almond butter
- Piece of your favorite fruit
- Carrot, celery, and/ or cucumber sticks with hummus
- Unsalted gluten-free crackers such as rice crackers with guacamole or hummus
- Kale chips
- Green vegetable juice
- Any green smoothie

Lunch Ideas: The ideal midday munch will be 70 percent vegetables, preferably raw, such as greens, broccoli, carrots, bell peppers, tomatoes, cucumbers, and beets. This will make it much easier to transition to all smoothies, all the time the following week. You can then fill the other 30 percent in with other plant foods, such as cooked chickpeas, gluten-free grains such as rice or quinoa, baked sweet potato, or steamed fish. Think salad drizzled with lemon juice and fresh herbs, chickpeas and vegetables seasoned with turmeric, ginger, and cumin, lentil soup, grain, and/or kale salad with almonds and cranberries

Dinner Ideas: Increase the vegetable ratio to 80 percent and fill the remainder in with grains, legumes, and lentils. If you don't want to spend a lot of time prepping, stick to the one bowl method: Combine 1 cup of cooked grains/beans/lentils, 1 cup of greens such as spinach or kale, 1 cup of vegetables such as steamed broccoli, avocado, hemp or chia seeds, or seaweed and ¼ cup of protein such as cubed white chicken or flaked salmon.

Other one bowl combos:

- Grilled portobello mushroom cap, brown rice, pine nuts, spinach, fresh Italian herbs, chopped tomato
- Steamed kale sprinkled with sunflower seeds and tossed in lemon juice and tofu mixed with brown rice or quinoa
- Steamed salmon with fresh herbs, lemon, and bok choy over millet
- Vegetable curry with brown rice and cashews
- Broccoli soup splashed with lemon
- Black bean salad with quinoa, avocado, and salsa
- Barley, walnuts, mushrooms, celery, carrots, and tomato paste

Two-Week Full-Body Cleanse Menu

Look for a balance of fiber, protein, and flavor to keep you energized all day. The important thing is to mimic a regular eating plan with breakfast, lunch, and dinner-type smoothies.

Wake-Up Call: Start with two 8-ounce glasses of water when you first wake up, adding a couple of tablespoons of protein powder if you need an extra boost of energy.

Breakfast: Any breakfast smoothie from the Recipe Box (page 221) plus a glass of water.

Make It to Lunch Snack: Iced or hot green or herbal tea plus a glass of water.

Post Lunch/Physical Activity: A tall glass of coconut water.

Lunch: Any lunch smoothie from the Recipe Box (page 221) plus a glass of water.

Midday Slump Snack: Any smoothie variation from the Master Green Smoothie section of the Recipe Box (page 221) plus a glass of water.

After-Work Drink: 2 glasses of plain or flavored water (see Water Flavorings, page 132).

Dinner: Any dinner smoothie from the Recipe Box (page 221) plus a glass of water

Night-time Munchies Snack: Any happy hour smoothie from the Recipe Box (page 221) plus a glass of water.

Post-Cleanse Clean-Up Menu

Days 1 to 3: Eat only vegetables, fruits, nuts, seeds, lentils, plant-based oils, and seasonings. Include one Master Green Smoothie variation (page 224).

Day 4: Introduce white fish, legumes, beans, and grains such as brown rice, quinoa, and oats; go easy on the salt. Include one Master Green Smoothie variation.

Day 5: Add eggs or soy (such as tofu or edamame) to the menu. Include one Master Green Smoothie variation.

Day 6: Add some lean meat such as chicken or pork. Include one Master Green Smoothie variation.

Day 7: Add a slice of whole-grain bread or 2 ounces of whole grain pasta to the menu. Include one Master Green Smoothie variation.

14 Quick Tip Steps to a New You

1. Be present. That means checking in with yourself and acknowledging how you're feeling physically and emotionally.

2. Journaling is a great way to "cleanse" your soul and relieve yourself of mental and emotional stress.

3. Give yourself an inner cleanse by letting go of something negative that has been holding you back. This may involve finding the half-full aspect of the glass or perhaps forgiving someone you have held a grudge against.

4. Restore yourself and rejuvenate your resolve daily with these touchstones:

   • I cleanse because my body and mind deserve rest.

   • I cleanse because I want to nourish myself with healing foods every day that satisfy and nurture my mind, body, and soul.

   • I cleanse because I deserve to feel vibrancy, love, peace, and joy in my life.

   • I cleanse because I can let go of all that I no longer need.

   • I cleanse because I live in the moment.

   • I cleanse because it's a gift I give myself.

   • I cleanse because I love and accept myself completely.

5. If the above smacks too much of self-love, try to invigorate your spirit by committing a bit of poetry to memory. Try this doggerel about spiritual renewal by William Butler Yeats:

   > *"The friends that have I do it wrong*
   > *Whenever I remake a song,*
   > *Should know what issue is at stake:*
   > *It's myself that I remake."*

6. Clear the clutter and clear your mind. Compulsive hoarding, a mental health disorder characterized by accumulation of excessive clutter, may affect up to 2 million Americans. But most of us are noncompulsive hoarders at heart: those jeans you fit into three years ago and you're sure you will fit into again, the drawing of a moose your child made in first grade, every book you have ever bought, the CDs from when you were briefly in an alterna-punk-hip hop jag, the "Home Sweet Gnome"

pillow you won at the Renaissance Faire…. But before you start sweeping through the debris of your life like a human tornado, make a plan. The key is to not feel overwhelmed, so focus on one room or even one area a day or week or month—whatever schedule works for you.

7. Breathe new life into yourself. The breath has a direct connection to the mind and is one of the fastest ways to settle the mind. Sit comfortably in a darkened room, hands on your lap with thumb and forefinger of each hand touching; close your eyes and inhale through your nose for a count of three, then exhale through the mouth for a count of five. Continue for three minutes.

8. If possible, try and close your eyes when you're feeling down. A 10-minute power nap can be enough to revive your spirit.

9. Meditate. At the core of this mental discipline is the goal to focus and eventually quiet your mind, setting free your awareness. But you don't have to spend all your vacations dressed in orange and living in an ashram or even ever say "ohm" to get started. Find a phrase or word that soothes you. This is your "mantra." Then sit comfortably on the ground, close your eyes, and recite your mantra in a steady rhythm, either in your head or out loud. Or, even easier, count your breath from 1 through 10, then begin again at 1. Continue for three minutes.

10. Leave at least one window open as often as possible. The fresh air will clear the room and your mind.

11. Tweak your daily routine by doing three things in a different order or one new thing every day. The breakup of your usual pattern keeps your mind refreshed.

12. Make social media your detective and get in touch with an old friend. Sometimes the surest path to a new you is reconnect-

ing with an old version of yourself by rebuilding bonds with someone you knew way back when.

13. Say no. No at work, no to friends, no to your family. Learning this short two-letter word can be extremely mentally freeing.

14. Spread the joy. Passing on a kind word (telling the cashier you like their earrings) or a thoughtful act (bringing a stressed colleague a flower) can lift your own spirit and actually make you think better about yourself.

WATCH OUT FOR

Swishy smoothie belly. You're drinking a lot of liquids. To offset feeling bloated, go to the toilet even when you don't think that you have to go. The more you release, the lighter you will feel.

Obsession. Yes, it's important to follow the basic guidelines of the cleanse, but you can become too focused on being absolutely pure with your food, which will inevitably lead to becoming uptight and judgmental—which is definitely not what the Two-Week Full-Body Cleanse is about. Relax. You're cleansing, not saving the world from destruction.

Pinterest. Instagram. Food magazines. Cooking shows. Samples at Whole Foods. Seriously, you don't want to go there.

Day 3. It's a killer. Try this tip from a group of Greenster women who swear it gets them over any hump: Watch some raw footage on films cheering the whole foods movement to stay motivated. Put the following titles on your list:

Fat, Sick, and Nearly Dead

Food Matters

Food, Inc.

Vegucated

Hungry for Change

Fathead

Ingredients

American Meat

Forks Over Knives

Farmageddon

Feeling like you can do this forever? You probably can, but you shouldn't unless you're a nutritionist and truly know how to balance your green smoothies.

THE PAYOFF

- You're not going to be able to avoid feeling a little loopy-headed during the cleanse at first, so make it work for you. Use the initial foggy symptoms of your cleanse as your all-purpose, get-out-of-jail-free card to explain why you made a mistake at work, why you lost to your partner at Bananagrams, why you forgot your aunt's birthday.
- You now know you're stronger than you thought. The sense of accomplishment that comes with finishing a two-week green smoothie cleanse makes you feel like you can take on the world—or at least negotiate for a better life insurance plan.
- You did it once so you know you can do it again. Extra payoff? Your body as well as your mind will hold a memory of the cleanse, so the next time (because once you have mastered it, there will always be a next time) will be easier.
- You feel superior to people who need solid food to survive.

CHAPTER SIXTEEN

Smoothie Sailing

You can't make an omelet without breaking eggs, and you can't make a green smoothie without the occasional mishap. Sure, it seems that as long as you avoid throwing in capers or anchovies, it's almost impossible to screw up making a green smoothie: Toss some leafy greens and fruit in a blender with some liquid and other goodies, press blend, and *insto! presto!* In a few minutes, you have a delish, nutrish drink.

But no matter how impressive your Greenster credentials, there will be times when you will be distracted and add too much protein into the mix or neatly pack up your liquid meal in a container to keep you sustained for a day of cleansing only to leave the bottle in your car and come back to a crime scene with bits of green smoothie exploded in every possible crack and crevice of your auto's interior.

Luckily, most mishaps can be salvaged and some can even be prevented with a little planning and know-how. Treat this chapter as your go-to fix-it reference to smooth over common green smoothie cleanse pitfalls. Drink up and learn.

Smooth It Over

How to blend it better and fix your smoothie mix-ups fast.

The Mix-Up: You didn't have time to cut, chop, and slice all the ingredients for your green smoothie, so you just left a few things out.

It ended up tasting just OK and you're pretty sure that you may have missed out on adding some of the key nutrients. You're thinking next time you're in a rush, it might be better to opt for a premade drink.

The Fix-Up: First, relax—it's food and it's good-for-you food, so your health profile will survive the ingredient gaps. Buying a drink is more likely to make you deficient in key vitamins while loading up on sugar. To fill up the flavor holes, make sure that you always have one of these three all-purpose tasty ingredients on hand (only add one): dark chocolate, bananas, berries.

Blend It Better Next Time: All it takes is a little prep to turn smoothie making into child's play (bonus, all that chopping counts as exercise). First, think big: Don't slice and dice for just one smoothie. Do a super shop and buy enough for a month of green smoothies. Then cut everything up, as smaller pieces (including greens) makes it easier to blend straight from frozen—but don't peel your ingredients (see Slap Me Some Skin, page 36). Freeze in separate portion bags (yes, it takes more bags, but it makes them easier to work with in the long run) and use as needed. Depending on the strength of your blender, you shouldn't have to defrost the ingredients. (If buying frozen fruit, be aware that purees often have added sugar.) You can make a green smoothie in seconds and you won't have to worry about your produce going bad. In a less-than-ideal world—i.e., the one where you have no time at all—you can blend and freeze your complete green smoothie in advance. In theory and reality, a green smoothie is best consumed asap after blending. If you do need to freeze it, store it in a thin, airtight freezer-proof glass container, filled to the brim, to reduce oxidation.

The Mix-Up: You added all of your ingredients and the blender is grinding slower than a wet weekend.

The Fix-Up: Add more liquid in small amounts until things get moving again.

Blend It Better Next Time: There's actually an order and a timing to adding green smoothie ingredients to the blender to keep things moving smoothly: 1) liquid base, 2) soft fruits, 3) harder and/or frozen fruits and/or vegetables. 4) Now add: leafy greens; blend again for a few seconds if you have a superduper blender and for as long as 3 minutes if you're working with a more basic model. 5) Add: Nuts/nut butters/ seeds. 6) Finally, put in any powder add-ins. Blend just until smooth. If using protein powder, the less blending at this point, the better, as the protein will transform into a wallpaper paste consistency if aerated too long. Add more liquid if needed. Studies show that keeping your smoothie on the thick side can make you feel fuller more quickly and for longer than a more liquid smoothie.

The Mix-Up: Your blender is making a horrible grinding sound that would send you straight to your mechanic if it came from your car.

The Fix-Up: Take everything out and strain the liquid smooth again. Chances are you left a pit in a piece of fruit.

Blend It Better Next Time: You could invest in a better smoothie blender (see the Mix-Up on using a food processor, page 207). But you still need to keep an eye out for the pits of certain fruits as they contain toxic elements (see Slap Me Some Skin on page 36 for which ones are safe to ingest).

The Mix-Up: There's a thick brownish scum on top of your green smoothie.

The Fix-Up: Blender blades work overtime to combine the produce and the water. The superfast speed can create an unappealing brackish foam as more air is added to the smoothie and oxidizes (a fancy way of saying air is mixed with another substance). Overripe bananas and some greens/fruit combos can also cause the bad brownish pond water look (remember your kindergarten painting lesson—red + green = brown) while milk and watery produce like frozen spinach and melons can make things bubbly. Try to shake (or stir) it out or simply skim the top. A splash of orange juice stirred in might also neutralize the primordial aspect of the smoothie, while thickeners like avocado, coconut flakes, or nut butters can help stabilize the lather.

Blend It Better Next Time: Blend at a lower speed or pulse. If you're short on time, then go with high speed, but blend for less time. The longer and more powerfully your blend, the more foam. Adding half the liquid before and the remaining after the other ingredients are completely blended can also help reduce froth.

The Mix-Up: You forgot to put the lid on the blender and sprayed green smoothie all over your kitchen, hair, and clothes. Or you left it in a warm car and it exploded into 1,000 random stains.

The Fix-Up: Ugh. It happens. Cleaning up smoothie spills of any size can be pretty challenging—the ingredients seem to be full of naturally staining properties. The key is to move quickly. Start with the most absorbent material: rugs, ceilings, walls. Scoop up any excess, blot the leftovers with a paper towel, and finally mix 1 teaspoon of vinegar with 1 cup of warm water and apply to the area. Let the stain soak in the cleaning solution for about 2 minutes and then begin blotting it using a clean white (so as not to leave dye stains) cloth. You might need to reapply some of the vinegar solution. Finally, when most of the stain is gone, pour a glass of water over the area and dry thoroughly.

Blend It Better Next Time: Work in an easier-to-clean (or, at least, paint over) station. If you're leaving your smoothie in the car, make sure it's in a cooler with an ice pack.

The Mix-Up: You love smoothies, but hate the blender clean-up.

The Fix-Up: Let the blender do the hard work for you. Immediately after pouring your smoothie into a glass, add warm water and a drop of washing-up liquid to the blender jar and blend on high for 30 seconds.

Blend It Better Next Time: If the blender is splotched in smoothie stains, mix 1 teaspoon of baking soda with 1 cup of warm water in the blender jar, pulse for 2 minutes, and then leave it to soak (with the cover on) overnight.

The Mix-Up: You always seem to make too much or too little green smoothie.

The Fix-Up: Freeze what you don't use. If you need more, thin it out with a protein or calorie-rich liquid such as milk, coconut water, or fruit juice.

Blend It Better Next Time: The general measurement is every 1 to 2 cups of liquid (depending on how thick you like your green smoothies) = 1 smoothie.

The Mix-Up: You forgot about your green smoothie that was blending on high and answered the phone. When you returned 5 minutes later (OK, maybe it was 10), the smoothie had transformed into an inedible, thin, brown slush.

The Fix-Up: You can try adding lemon juice or pineapple or anything with citric acid, which may help neutralize some of the oxidization. But taste it first—it may be one of those situations when it looks worse than it tastes.

Blend It Better Next Time: Depending on the power of your blender, a typical green smoothie should take no more than 1 to 3 minutes to whip up. So if you tend toward culinary ADD, think about pulsing your smoothies so you don't overblend them.

The Mix-Up: You just realized that you'll need to lug your daily supply of green smoothies around wherever you go.

The Fix-Up: If you can't store your green smoothie stash in a fridge, you don't need to buy a special carrying case. If you're just going to and from work and have access to a fridge there, any nonbreakable container with a tight-fitting lid will do. If you have to keep your smoothies with you, then recycle an old plastic jug and fill it with the drink (this is a short-term solution; for the long-term, you'll want to ensure the plastic is BPA free) and bundle it with a freezer pack.

Blend It Better Next Time: Investing in an all-temperature, insulated thermos is worth it to keep your smoothie cold and fresh-tasting. They're available in several sizes so you can customize them to your daily needs. On the plus size, carting the extra weight around can help you build muscle!

The Mix-Up: You'll have to take out a small loan to finance a two-week green smoothie cleanse.

The Fix-Up: Much produce is transported before it's actually ripe, so you may actually sometimes be better off picking up marked-down produce that's a little old and bruised. There's almost always a bunch of brown, spotted bananas that look past their prime but are actually at the ripening tipping point when they offer the most nutritionally. Buy in bulk and freeze what you're not planning to use right away (peel bananas and chop everything to blending size first).

Blend It Better Next Time: Think outside the fresh box. Canned and sometimes frozen produce is less expensive than fresh, is more likely to be discounted with coupons, and, as long as no salt or sugar has been added, can be just as healthy (see Spoiler Alert, page 38). Other penny-pinching moves: Make your own add-ins (see Make It, Don't Buy It, page 82), dilute juices and milks with a little water to get more liquid for your buck, buy produce in season as it tends to be a little less expensive (or grow your own—even cheaper!), and stop buying expensive supplements and energy/protein drinks as you don't need them.

The Mix-Up: You don't want to get a new blender when your old one works perfectly fine—except for making green smoothies, which come out more like hacked greens.

The Fix-Up: If it ain't broke, why fix it? But be prepared to put a little more effort into your prep work. If the smoothie ingredients are too thick, the blade tends to spin too fast and keep everything pushed out to the sides and not actually blended. So you'll need to chop everything extra fine and small and possibly work in batches to get it as chunk free as possible.

Blend It Better Next Time: A green smoothie should in theory be simply a bing, bang, boom drink—throw the ingredients in, blend, and voilà! If your blender cannot handle the bing and the bang, add the liquid first to keep things loose. Then, instead of one sustained blend, try pulsing each ingredient after adding it. Sometimes short bursts of power tend to stir up some of the bits and pieces that sneak underneath the blades. Also, try freezing the cut fruit before, which may help prevent it from getting mushed and mucking up the blades. If your blender has one, use the ice-crushing blade, which is better equipped to deal with fortified ingredients. When blending, start at the lowest speed and gradually work your way higher. Your blender will let you know when it's time to stop, as it will begin emitting a low-pitched whine. Immediately drop one speed lower. As a last resort, tip the blender at an angle and shake forcefully or use a chopstick to shift things around between pulses. Know, however, that however much prep work and time you put in to working your old blender, your green smoothie will never live up to its name unless you're using a machine that is 1,000 watts or more.

The Mix-Up: You used a food processor instead of a blender, and now you have a choppie instead of a smoothie.

The Fix-Up: A food processor or even a basic blender isn't going to give you the smooth finish of a more powerful blender. But your green smoothie will still taste fine; it will just require more chewing.

Blend It Better Next Time: You can make a green smoothie in any kind of blender. It may take longer or have a smaller capacity, but any machine will do the job. If it can't handle the frozen produce, let the fruit and vegetables defrost for an hour before blending. However, if green smoothies are going to be a daily part of your life, it's worth it to bite the cost and invest in a lean green smoothie–blending machine. Your blender is going to be your ultimate power tool and you want one that can do the job. A high-power blender will take less time to make the smoothie and it will blend the ingredients more efficiently with less prep time. You may even save money in the long run as the wear and tear green smoothies can place on a blender not up to the job can quickly send it to the junk heap. The four-star general of blenders is a Vita-Mix, which works like Robo Cop, crushing frozen whole fruit, greens, and ice all in one batch without breaking down. It isn't cheap but it will last for years. However, any blender in the 1,000-watt and above range will get the job done.

Sip It

How to turn a smoothie fail into a lip-smacking success with these recipes to fix your disasters.

The Awful Awful: Your green smoothie tastes like it should be served with nachos.

Lip-Smacking Solution: While avocado is an ideal go-to ingredient, you can get too much of this good thing. Don't use more than ¼ of an avocado to avoid it overwhelming the flavor of your smoothie. If it does end up tasting like guacamole, try adding some more leafy greens and liquid.

The Awful Awful: No matter what ingredients you use, your green smoothies taste disgusting.

Lip-Smacking Solution: This may be a case of equipment (or rather, equipment cleaner) malfunction rather than something lacking in the smoothie recipes or ingredients. Take your blender completely apart, including the gasket from the blade. Chances are there's a gunky buildup that is affecting not only the taste but also the hygiene of your smoothies. To thoroughly clean the blades, fully immerse them in 3 cups of water mixed with 4 tablespoons of baking soda and 1 cup of vinegar (use a tall container, as the vinegar/baking soda combo creates an explosive reaction—be prepared for lots of foam). Leave to soak overnight. When reassembling the blender, rub 1 tablespoon of vegetable oil on the blender gasket to keep it flexible (the gasket is the piece that separates the jug from the base). If you have dirt buildup around your control buttons, clean it with a Q-tip dipped in rubbing alcohol. It will lift the gunk away from the hard-to-clean crevices and evaporate quickly so it won't damage your electrical base.

In the future, before adding ingredients to the jug, make sure the blender is tightly closed at the bottom to prevent liquid from leaking out and mucking up the works. If you don't have time to give the blender jug and blade a thorough cleaning after making your smoothie, disassemble them and put them in warm, soapy water mixed with 1 tablespoon of vinegar and a couple of drops of dishwashing soap to soak. The extra step may seem like a hassle, but if you skip it, you'll be mixing dirt and old food bits into your kale-berry smoothie, which doesn't sound very delicious or nutritious.

The Awful Awful: You hate following a recipe. But your smoothies are more miss than hit.

Lip-Smacking Solution: There are three types of smoothie makers in the world: 1) people who can chuck everything but the kitchen sink into the blender and somehow produce a delicious smoothie, 2) people who are scared to add so much as an extra parsley sprig if it isn't listed in the recipe, and 3) people who think they fall into the first category but are better off following a recipe. If you're adding whatever sounds good to your smoothie but the results are undrinkable, it's time to get back to basics and follow a recipe.

This doesn't mean you can never wander from the path of measurements again. But a good chef is like a trophy-winning coach: You know your ingredients and have a sense of their flavors, moisture, texture, and even weight, which means that you can make substitutions without second-guessing yourself. However, if you're more a bumbling Inspector Clouseau than a master Hercule Poirot in the kitchen, then here's your cheat list for ingredient subs. Each ingredient can be indiscriminately exchanged for any other item in each group in the list that follows:

Fresh/Frozen: Most fresh ingredients can be subbed with the frozen version of the same ingredient (frozen blueberries for fresh blueberries, for example), and, certainly in the case of fruit but also some vegetables will often taste better than the fresh version (see Spoiler Alert, page 38). Just take care to add a bit more liquid so the consistency doesn't get too icy and thick. If you go the other way and use fresh instead of frozen, add less liquid and a bit more ice.

Fruit

- Berries of any kind
- Strawberries, raspberries, or peaches
- Mango, papaya, or pineapple
- Peaches, apricots, or nectarines
- Acai berry, cherries, or blueberries
- Kiwi, fresh strawberries with a squeeze of lime juice, or green grapes
- Apples or pears
- Apricots, pluots, peaches, or nectarines
- Bananas, mango, or papaya
- Plums, cherries, or nectarines

Add-Ins

- Coconut water ice cubes or regular water ice cubes
- Carob chips or bittersweet chocolate chips
- Cacao/cocoa nibs (toast whole cocoa beans and crumble) or semisweet chocolate chips
- 1 ounce bittersweet chocolate, ⅔ ounce unsweetened chocolate, and 2 teaspoons of granulated organic sugar, or 1 ounce semisweet chocolate and ¼ teaspoon cocoa powder
- Allspice or ¼ teaspoon ground cinnamon and ½ teaspoon ground cloves
- Gingerroot, ground ginger, or (for a sweeter variation) chopped crystallized ginger
- Ground allspice, cloves, nutmeg, or mace
- Lemon juice, two-thirds the amount of lime juice (so if recipe calls for 1 teaspoon lemon juice, use ⅔ teaspoon lime juice) or half the amount of malt vinegar (so if recipe calls for 1 teaspoon lemon juice, subsitute ½ teaspoon malt vinegar)
- Apple cider vinegar, lemon juice, tart apple juice, or white vinegar
- Goji berries, dried cranberries, or currants

Nuts, Grains, and Seeds

- Sesame seeds, pumpkin seeds, cashews, or half the amount of tahini (so if recipe calls for 1 cup of seeds or cashews, use ½ cup tahini)
- Brazil nuts, macadamia nuts, almonds, or raw coconut meat
- Almonds, hazelnuts, or shelled pistachios
- Pecans, hickory nuts, or walnuts
- Walnuts, cashews, hazelnuts, or almonds

- Any nut butter or seed butter
- Chia seeds or flaxseeds
- Amaranth, millet, or quinoa

Liquids
- Chai concentrate or the same amount of chilled black or chai tea plus 1 tablespoon agave syrup per cup of liquid
- Cashew juice or 5 parts apple juice to 1 part lemon juice
- Coconut milk, 1 part coconut cream with 4 parts low-fat milk, or 1 part coconut flavoring with 8 parts whole milk
- Coconut water, or 1 part coconut milk and 1 part water
- Soy milk, hemp milk, almond milk, rice milk, or grain milk
- Kefir, buttermilk, yogurt, or Greek yogurt

Sweeteners
- Agave syrup, maple syrup, sweet apple cider, or ½ banana
- Honey, molasses, or maple syrup
- Vegetables
- Broccoli, broccoli rabe, or cauliflower
- Red cabbage, Napa cabbage, or green cabbage
- Carrots, parsnip, daikon, or celery
- Celery, fennel, bok choy, or jicama
  Pumpkin or butternut squash
- Chickpeas, great Northern beans, or lima beans

Leafy Greens
- Green cabbage, Savoy cabbage, or Napa cabbage
- Spinach, Swiss chard, or kale
- Bibb lettuce, Boston lettuce, butterhead, or red or green leaf lettuce

The Awful Awful: Something went horribly wrong and your green smoothie tastes like something you have to drink to prepare for a colonoscopy.

Lip-Smacking Solution: Nothing may have gone wrong—some recipes taste better on paper than in reality. You can salvage the drink by pouring half into a jar and refrigerating it to use as a base for tomorrow. Makeover what's left by adding fruit; the best picks to mask bad tastes are bananas and citrus, juice, sweetener, and ice.

Some secret ingredients for the future:

- Add ice cubes for extra froth.
- Add cider vinegar to give your smoothie a tangy zest.
- Add kombucha to make your smoothie a fizzy drink fest.
- Old fruit with brown spots will give your drink the sweetest taste.

The Awful Awful: You used frozen vegetables and fruit and the smoothie is thicker than *Family Guy's* Peter Griffin.

Lip-Smacking Solution: There's nothing wrong with substituting frozen for fresh as long as you compensate by using less ice and a little more liquid to keep the consistency smooth enough to sip. Less is always best when it comes to adding liquids, as it's easier to pour in more to liquefy a too-thick smoothie than thicken a drink that is too runny, as you risk overblending the main fruit and vegetable ingredients. However, if you accidentally overcompensate by adding too much extra liquid, readjust by throwing in the all-purpose banana or, if you don't want to add more sugar, an avocado, either of which will easily smooth things over.

The Awful Awful: You wanted to adjust the 60:40 ratio to amp up the greens but the result was as bitter as a bowl of chicory.

Lip-Smacking Solution: The all-purpose SOS (Save Our Smoothie) trio of banana, citrus, and/or avocado will take the edge off. Carrots and kohlrabi can also balance out bitterness while honey, vinegar, lemon, or lime juice will add a sweeter note. Before changing the ratio, get on intimate terms with your leafy greens to figure out which is the most likely culprit for bitterness. Taste as you add and if it makes your mouth pucker, find a milder substitute. Baby greens are also generally milder than mature greens.

The Awful Awful: The seeds didn't grind and your smoothie tasted more like a mouthful of grit.

Lip-Smacking Solution: For now, avocado or banana will add a touch of "cream" and bring all the flavors together. If your blender isn't powerful enough to pulverize seeds like flax, chia, or hemp, soak them in water, juice, or any liquid for a few hours first to soften them into a blendable pulpy mass. Yum. There's nothing much you can do about seeds from fruits like pomegranates or raspberries other than take the extra step and strain the drink for a smooth finish.

The Awful Awful: You added everything in the correct proportions but the smoothie is as tasteless and flabby as a piece of day-old gum.

Lip-Smacking Solution: Chances are the fruit was underripe. This tends to make the smoothie watery and has less than zero flavor. Next time, if there's no ready fruit, choose over-ready fruit. It may actually be better for you anyway (and certainly less expensive). Studies found that the amount of antioxidants in fruits grows as they get closer to spoiling.

The Awful Awful: You had some leftover salad from dinner last night and it ended up tasting like slimy swamp.

Lip-Smacking Solution: It feels tempting to raid your shelves and just chuck in every slightly wilted and best-by item of food that you have, but when you make leftovers that are on their last legs the main flavor, that is exactly how your green smoothie will taste. If it's really thick and brown, throw it away and try again. But if it is only this side of slush, try rejuvenating it up with some fresher stuff or the go-to SOS of banana, citrus, and/or avocado.

The Awful Awful: Your green smoothie flavors were not coming together so you kept stuffing things in. Now, instead of a couple cups of so-so green smoothie, you have a gallon of really horrid mush.

Lip-Smacking Solution: Get friendly with your spice rack—a sprinkle of cinnamon and a dash of nutmeg or even hot sauce can go a long way toward covering up some really bad flavor combos, as can the previously mentioned SOS of banana, citrus, or avocado.

The reality is, "the kitchen sink" is the not-to-take approach when making a smoothie. Some vegetables and fruit simply don't play nicely together and can actually turn a good smoothie bad. So more isn't going to be better. You won't get more nutrition out of one smoothie by piling in the ingredients for the simple reason that the results are usually so revolting that you'll have trouble finishing the drink, let alone have a great desire to make another one. If you're working off the cuff and not following a recipe, then always start your smoothie with a maximum of four ingredients: one kind of green leafy vegetable, one fruit, one liquid, and one add-in flavor. Then taste, taste, taste before adding anything else. The chefs who always lose on the cooking competitions are the ones who forget to dip their spoon in their own concoctions as they are putting them together. The light touch also means that the cleanse will be less likely to upset your digestive system.

The Awful Awful: The kale leaves are too tough to pulverize and they taste like a horrible cross between really strong beer and dirt.

Lip-Smacking Solution: If possible, keep on blending to pulverize as much as possible. Add some cored pineapple to balance out the strong taste. In the future, select a sweeter, less stringy kale. There are several varieties of kale: curly kale (deep green ruffled leaves, earthy, peppery flavor, and fibrous stalk), ornamental kale (also called salad Savoy, more tender and mild flavored), and dinosaur kale (dark blue-green leaves, delicate, almost sweet flavor). Also, use kale ASAP. The longer it's kept, the more bitter it becomes (within two days of purchase is a good standard to follow). Finally, if your blender starts to moan when put to work, then try chopping the kale leaves before adding them. Note the word "leaves"—they should be de-stemmed and de-ribbed, as these parts of the kale only add to the strong taste and make them tougher to blend. Alternate between adding a little kale at a time, blending between each addition.

The Awful Awful: The smoothie consistency was thinner than a super-model on a diet.

Lip-Smacking Solution: Throw in some instant heavy weights—creamy vegetables or fresh or frozen fruit like avocados or bananas, ice cubes, grains, nut butters, and tofu will all add to the smoothie's waistline. If your smoothies consistently tend to be on the runny side, then you may not be adding enough protein on a regular basis (see Add-Ins, page 211). Most adults would benefit from eating more than the RDA of 56 grams. The pluses go beyond muscles. Protein shrinks hunger and can help prevent obesity, diabetes, and heart disease. If you're on a multiday green smoothie cleanse, you especially need to bump up your protein intake. The fewer calories you consume, the more calories should come from protein. Get on the scale and add between 0.50 and 0.75 grams of protein per pound of body weight daily to preserve calorie-burning muscle mass.

The Awful Awful: The smoothie is tarter than a sour lemon.

Lip-Smacking Solution: Add something sweet. It doesn't have to be something from the Sweet Indulgences list (page 76). Mango, apple, and berries can also prevent a pucker up. If you're too heavy-handed with the sweet touch, add a teaspoon of lemon juice or soaked chia seeds to balance out the flavor. Next time, think about what fruits and vegetables you're using. Some are naturally sweeter or more peppery than others and may need to be balanced out in your overall 60:40 ratio. See Have It Your Way (page 59) for info on milder-tasting produce and How Sweet It Is (page 232) for a guaranteed sweet smoothie.

The Awful Awful: By the time you finish your daily quart of green smoothie, it has turned into a cup of brown sludge.

Lip-Smacking Solution: If you're a slow drinker, pour out 4 ounces of smoothie at a time to sip on and store the remainder in the refrigerator or a cooler to keep it tasting sweet and green. A teaspoon of lemon juice may also help preserve your smoothie's fresh appeal. The culprit may also be bananas, which rapidly turn drinks brown the longer they sit. If that's the case, a quick stir will help the taste, but there's nothing you can do about the unappealing appearance.

The Awful Awful: The temperature of the green smoothie is making your teeth ache.

Lip-Smacking Solution: While you want to keep your smoothie cold to avoid losing flavor and having the whole thing turn an ugly shade of brown, it isn't exactly a palate pleaser to try and down a frosty drink if you live in a cold clime. Don't heat it up—this is about keeping things raw. But you can stir in a little hot liquid to bring up the temperature. Shaking your smoothie vigorously will also take some of the chill out.

Strut It Out

Green smoothies may leave you feeling cleansed inside and out, but there are potentially rough(age) moments that can lead to some beautiful disasters. Forewarned is forearmed.

Indulge your vanity and check in with a mirror each and every time after drinking a green smoothie, unless green mustaches and green bits in the teeth are considered fashion statements in your neck of the woods. Drinking through a straw will help minimize the mess.

Mason jars as cups are must-have accessories when on a green smoothie cleanse, as much for the way they instantly announce that you are on a cleanse as for the BPA-free glass. Just remember to put on the lid (you can have a second lid with a hole punched in it for a straw), or the green spillage all over your shirt will also turn you into a walking advertisement for green smoothies.

While green smoothies are great ways to fill you up, know that the room they take up in your stomach is not the only volume they will create. The ingredients tend to cause loud belly gurgles and belches. To turn down the tunes, sip slowly and chew the bits of green as much as possible. If you aren't on a cleanse, try eating a little protein before drinking to quiet stomach rumbles.

A green smoothie cleanse can initially make you dizzy, often at the most inopportune times, like a meeting with your boss. To avoid landing in their lap, make sure you add some protein to your smoothie before going to work.

Natural gas may be all the rage these days, but not when your body is producing it. To sidestep the stink, cut back on the fruit fiber in your smoothie and space out the drinks during the day so you are glugging less at each sitting. Another solution is to crack down on the amount of nuts, avocado, and other oil-based ingredients, as the triple-F food for thought is too much fat + too much fruit = too many farts. While you're waiting for the gas stage to pass, fill up on these fascinating fart facts:

- You may not be letting out as much air as you think. The average person on an average day breaks wind an average of 14 times. In measurable terms, this means they produce about ½ liter of farts.

- You are not off the hook if you're a woman—men and women are equal when it comes to passing gas.

- The average fart is composed of about 59 percent nitrogen, 21 percent hydrogen, 9 percent carbon dioxide, 7 percent methane, and 4 percent oxygen. Less than 1 percent of their makeup is hydrogen sulfide (what makes gas stink).

- Farts have been clocked at a speed of 10 feet per second.

Don't be surprised if what is coming out of your bottom end looks a lot like what you just drank a few hours ago. All the fiber in green smoothies wreaks havoc on your digestive tract initially (see page 139 for more on what a normal cleanse stool looks like). It will take a week or so for things to stabilize. To add some backbone to your bowels, whip up a Stop the Trots smoothie (page 237).

If your digestive engine is running the other way, drinking more water can help flush things out. The Stop the Clog Smoothie (page 237) will stop bowels from getting blocked up and causing bellyaches.

While green smoothies have a wide variety of ingredients, the fact that they all tend to come from the same food groups can sometimes make breath reek. A handful of parsley or mint in your green smoothie will keep you kissing sweet, or in a pinch, gargle with a cup of warm salty water for about 30 seconds.

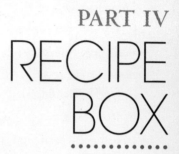

PART IV

RECIPE BOX

These recipes are for the perfectionist cook who must follow every measurement to the exact ⅛ teaspoon, the kitchen sink cook who throws in a bit of this and that, and every kind of cook in between. The point is, you can follow the instructions or switch, swap, and shimmy as desired.

A few housekeeping notes before you start blending:

- All recipes will make about 16 ounces.

- Refrigerate the smoothie if you are not drinking it immediately.

- Prep work will keep things smooth: Chop vegetables and fruit into small chunks before blending. Some people don't like the fibrous stem and ribs of green leafy vegetables and cut them out; others could care less. You'll know which camp you fall in after one sip.

- If you use frozen fruit, you may not need as much ice.

- If you have a mega-powered blender, you can add all the ingredients at the same time. If you have a base model, add the liquids, followed by the fruit and then the greens; throw in the extra vegetable and/or fruit, with add-ins last, pulsing for 30 seconds between each addition to ensure that your ingredients get blended. As the recipes become more complicated, add the ingredients in the order listed.

- Work your blender's buttons from slowest to fastest to gradually blend the ingredients.

- Always add ice last no matter what kind of blender you have as it may cause you to overblend, creating a watery drink.

MASTER GREEN SMOOTHIE (high-protein)

This is your all-purpose model: in essence, the perfect green smoothie. From here, the world is your green oyster as you can create endless variations with this basic recipe by using different greens, fruit, liquid, or including more add-ins.

- ½ cup liquid
- 1 fruit or 1 cup fruit
- 2 cups leafy greens
- ½ cup vegetable and/or 1 small or ½ cup fruit
- 1 add-in (optional)
- 1 to 2 tablespoons sweetener (optional)

Add water and/or ice depending if you want a more liquid or frostier drink.

INGREDIENT CHOICES

LIQUIDS

Water*

Coconut water

Soy milk

Rice milk

Nut milk

100% fruit juice

MAIN FRUIT

Avocados*

Bananas*

Blackberries

Blueberries

Mangoes

Peaches

Pineapples

Raspberries

Strawberries

LEAFY GREENS

Collard greens

Kale*

Romaine lettuce

Spinach*

Swiss chard

ADD-INS

2 tablespoons presoaked chia seeds

2 teaspoons ground cinnamon

¼ cup flaked or shredded unsweetened coconut

2 tablespoons presoaked flaxseed

1-inch chunk gingerroot

¼ cup lemon or lime juice

2 tablespoons nut butter*

¼ cup nuts*

¼ cup rolled oats

2 tablespoons spirulina

2 ounces tofu*

¼ cup yogurt*

SWEETENERS

Honey

2 Medjool dates*

Stevia*

ADDITIONAL VEGETABLES

Broccoli

Carrot*

1 small bunch lemon balm

1 small bunch mint

1 small bunch parsley*

ADDITIONAL FRUIT

Apple*

Lemon

Lime

Orange

Pear*

* Best base ingredients

MASTER GREEN SMOOTHIE VARIATIONS

Amp the vegetables by reversing the ratio to 60% leafy greens and 40% fruit.

20 YUMMY LIQUID/FRUIT/ADD-IN COMBOS

lemonade-strawberry

mango-banana

kiwi-berry-citrus

banana-pineapple

ginger-lemon-mint

blackberry-soy milk

pomegranate-blueberry

cranberry-lime juice

grape-lemon balm

cherry-strawberry

blueberry-tangerine-banana

banana-apple-raspberry

spirulina-blueberry

papaya-soy milk-banana

strawberry-banana-lemon-orange

lychee-coconut-banana

pineapple-banana-coconut

orange-banana-grapefruit

coconut-watermelon-lime-mint

pear-lime juice-mint

Make one week of All-Purpose Smoothies: Chop and freeze 21 bunches of green leafy vegetables (about 70 cups) and 35 small fruit (about 35 cups). This will give you a fast start to whatever kind of green smoothie you decide to whip up as you can toss them into the blender frozen and skip the ice.

Starter Newbie Smoothie: Use only spinach as your green leafy vegetable with 1) 100% apple juice-banana-strawberry, 2) 100% orange juice-banana-peach, 3) 100% orange juice-banana-mango, 4) 100% orange juice-banana-pineapple

THE SALADS-BORE-ME GREEN SMOOTHIE

coconut water

½ banana

½ mango

1 cup spinach

1 cup lettuce of choice

carrots

ginger

honey

GREENSTER PRACTICALLY NO FRUIT SMOOTHIE

water

½ avocado

1 cup spinach

1 cup kale

½ cucumber

3 basil leaves

½ lime

½ small bunch parsley

½ small bunch mint

Breakfast Green Smoothies

Everything you need for your wake-up call (except the caffeine).

MORE-THAN-GRAPEFRUIT SMOOTHIE

¼ cup water

¼ cup 100% citrus juice

1 small whole apple

2 cups kale

4 ribs celery

1 cucumber

1 ruby red grapefruit

PROTEIN-FIBER MORNING POWER PUNCH
(high-protein)

1 cup soy milk

½ cup other nut milk

1 banana

½ cup mustard greens

½ cup kale

2 cups spinach

½ green apple

½ cup grapes

1 small pear

¼ cup blueberries

¼ cup blackberries

2 tablespoons protein powder

1 tablespoon presoaked chia
seeds

1 tablespoon ground
flaxseeds

1 tablespoon nut, coconut, or
avocado oil

pinch of turmeric

1 tablespoon stevia or agave
nectar

3 to 4 cups ice

ALMOST CUP OF JOE SMOOTHIE

½ cup non-caffeinated green
tea

1 frozen banana

1 cup chicory

1 cup mild lettuce, such as
Bibb, Boston, or butterhead

2 tablespoons hazelnut butter
(or another nut butter)

2 tablespoons maple syrup
if you usually add sugar to
your coffee

A splash of your choice milk
if you usually have cream in
your coffee. Otherwise add
water as needed.

GOLDILOCKS SMOOTHIE (high-protein)

1 cup coconut water

1 banana

2 cups baby spinach

1 cup fresh or ½ cup dried
berries of choice

4 tablespoons presoaked
steel-cut oats

2 tablespoons presoaked
flaxseeds

1 teaspoon ground cinnamon

2 tablespoons maple syrup

2 tablespoons protein powder

VERMONT STACK (high-protein)

1 cup water

1 cup blueberries

1 cup spinach

1 cup mild lettuce, like butterhead, Bibb, or Boston

1 banana

¼ cup ground amaranth or cooked millet

1 tablespoon ground flaxseed

2 tablespoons protein powder

2 tablespoons maple syrup

1 teaspoon vanilla extract

½ cup kefir, yogurt, or cottage cheese

KISS: KEEP IT SIMPLE SMOOTHIE

1 cup nut milk

2 cups spinach

1 banana

THE NO TIME FOR BREAKFAST SMOOTHIE (high-protein)

1 cup water

2 bananas

1 head green leaf lettuce

1 cup kale

1 mango

½ cup strawberries

1 tablespoon ground flaxseeds

2 tablespoons protein powder

sprinkle of ground nutmeg

Lunch

A salad bar of green smoothies to keep you full until dinner.

RANCH HOUSE SALAD (high-protein)

1 cup water

¼ avocado

1 cup romaine lettuce

1 cup spinach

2 carrots

½ onion

1 tomato

1 cup Greek yogurt

1 garlic clove

1 teaspoon chives

1 teaspoon dill

dash of salt and pepper

SUPER GREEN GODDESS (high-protein)

½ cup 100% white grape
  juice

½ cup water

½ avocado

2 cups kale leaves

1 cup spinach leaves

1 green apple

1 pear

1 cup green grapes

½ bunch parsley

1 tablespoon spirulina or
  chlorella powder

¼ cup pumpkin seeds

CHOPPED SALAD

1 cup water

½ avocado

2 cups romaine lettuce

1 cup red cabbage

1 cucumber

2 radishes (optional)

1 large Fuji apple

1 Asian pear

1 mango

¼ cup hazelnuts

¼ cup pomegranate seeds

2 tablespoon nut or avocado
  oil

½ tablespoon honey

1½ tablespoons finely
  chopped onion

2 tablespoons cider vinegar

WALDORF SALAD (high-protein)

1 cup water

1 cup collards

1 cup mild lettuce, such as
  butterhead, Bibb, or Boston

1 red apple

½ cup red grapes

½ cup celery

¼ cup parsley

¼ cup walnuts

1 tablespoon lemon juice

¼ cup yogurt or kefir

dash salt and pepper

SPINACH STRAWBERRY SALAD (high-protein)

½ cup water

½ cup 100% cranberry juice

2 cups kale

½ banana

1 mango

1 cup strawberries

1 carrot

1 beet

¼ cup walnuts or pecans

¼ cup mint

2 tablespoons protein powder

2 tablespoons balsamic vinegar

Dinner

Take-out dinners that don't require ordering in.

FAST MCFOOD LOVER'S SMOOTHIE (high-protein)

Don't be put off by the brownish red color.

½ cup 100% orange juice

1 cup nut butter

½ cup water

1 banana

2 cups Swiss chard leaves

2 cups beets

½ cup strawberries

½ cup raspberries

¼ cup ground flaxseed

1 tablespoon raw cacao powder or cocoa

NACHOS BAR FOOD

½ cup water

½ cup 100% tomato juice

1 avocado

1 cup spinach

1 cup cabbage

¼ cup pineapple

½ banana

1 peach

1 tomato

1 tablespoon pumpkin seeds

1 tablespoon cilantro

1 tablespoon lime juice

1 teaspoon raw cacao powder or cocoa

dash of ground cinnamon

LEFTOVERS SMOOTHIE (high-protein)

½ cup water

½ cup any nut milk/cow milk/100% fruit juice about to hit its best-by date

2 cups any greens you need to get rid of

1 banana or avocado hitting just the other side of ripeness

1 cup soft fruit heading toward mushiness (such as strawberries, blueberries, peaches, apricots, nectarines)

any herbs starting to wilt (such as parsley, mint, cilantro, dill, thyme)

2 tablespoons lemon and/or lime juice

1 inch gingerroot

1 teaspoon ground cardamom

2 tablespoons honey or stevia

ASIAN STIR-FRY

1 cup water

1 cup bok choy

1 cup tatsoi

1 Fuji apple or Asian pear

½ red or orange bell pepper

2 broccoli stalks

½ bunch cilantro

½ garlic clove

2 tablespoons lime juice

1 tablespoon honey

CHINESE TAKE-OUT (high-protein)

1 cup water

1 small clementine

1 cup bok choy

1 cup mustard greens

1 cup spinach

½ cup edamame

2 ounces tofu

½ cup cooked brown rice

½ cucumber

2 carrots

1 garlic clove

½ inch gingerroot

1 tablespoon peanut butter

1 tablespoon honey

1 teaspoon soy sauce

BESTO PESTO SMOOTHIE (high-protein)

1 cup water

1 cup arugula

1 cup spinach

¼ avocado

½ cup basil

½ cup broccoli rabe

2 garlic cloves

½ cup precooked millet

2 tablespoons pine nuts

1 tablespoon wheat germ

¼ cup plain ricotta cheese

1 teaspoon balsamic vinegar

1 teaspoon red wine vinegar

MASALA CURRY SMOOTHIE (high-protein)

1 cup coconut water

1 cup 100% mango juice

½ avocado

1 banana

1 cup mustard greens

1 cup spinach

1 mango

⅓ cup unsweetened coconut flakes or shreds

1 tablespoon presoaked chia seeds

1 tablespoon honey

½ teaspoon garam masala

½ teaspoon ground cinnamon

½ cup yogurt

Snack and Kid-Friendly

VERY BERRY SMOOTHIE (high-protein)

¼ cup 100% orange juice

¼ cup 100% pomegranate juice

1 cup water

1 banana

2 cups spinach

1 cup blueberries

½ cup raspberries

2 small beets

1 teaspoon lime juice

1 tablespoon chopped mint (optional)

2 tablespoons stevia or honey

¼ cup yogurt

GREEN CHAI LATTE (high-protein)

1½ cups almond milk

1 banana

2 cups spinach

1 celery rib

¼ cup parsley

1 large pitted Medjool date

1 tablespoon ground flaxseed

1 inch gingerroot

1 tablespoon ground cinnamon

2 teaspoons ground cloves

2½ tablespoons ground cardamom

2 teaspoons ground nutmeg

2 teaspoons ground allspice

PEANUT BUTTER AND JELLY SMOOTHIE (high-protein)

½ cup water

½ cup nut milk

1 banana

1 cup green leaf lettuce

1 cup red leaf lettuce

1 cup strawberries

1 tablespoon peanut butter

3 Medjool dates

1 tablespoon ground flaxseed

HOW SWEET IT IS SMOOTHIE

1 cup 100% pomegranate juice

½ cup water

1 banana

2 cups Napa cabbage

1 cup seedless green grapes

1 pear

1 cup pineapple

1 mango

2 teaspoons lemon juice

1 teaspoon wheat germ

1 tablespoon pumpkin seeds

¼ cup chopped dark chocolate

2 pieces crystallized ginger

2 sprigs mint

dash of ground cinnamon

CHOCOLATE LOVER'S SMOOTHIE (high-protein)

1 ½ cups nut milk

2 bananas

1 cup chicory

1 cup spinach

¼ cup strawberries

2 tablespoons almond butter

4 ounces dark chocolate

2 tablespoons cacao powder or cocoa

1 tablespoon wheat germ or ground flaxseed

1 teaspoon balsamic vinegar

Happy Hour

All these cocktails are missing—besides the alcohol—are little paper umbrellas!

VIRGIN MARY

1 cup 100% tomato juice

½ cup water

1 cup radicchio

1 cup Savoy cabbage

¼ avocado

1 large cucumber, preferably English (seedless)

3 ribs celery, divided (reserve 1 to serve)

1 broccoli stalk

1 inch gingerroot

½ teaspoon fresh grated horseradish root or 1 drained teaspoon horseradish from a jar (optional)

3 drops Worcestershire sauce (optional)

1 teaspoon lemon or lime juice

EGGNOG (high-protein)

1 cup soy or rice milk

2 cups Napa cabbage

1 banana

1 teaspoon vanilla extract

¼ cup Greek yogurt

¼ teaspoon rum extract (optional)

¼ teaspoon nutmeg

GRASSHOPPER (high-protein)

1½ cups almond or rice milk

1 banana

1 cup chicory or endive

1 cup mild lettuce such as
Bibb, Boston, or butterhead

1 teaspoon stevia

2 ounces dark chocolate,
melted

1 teaspoon chlorella
(optional)

1 teaspoon chopped
mint leaves (preferably
peppermint)

TROPICAL DAIQUIRI

1 cup water

½ cup 100% passion fruit or
pomegranate juice

1 banana

2 cups spinach

5 strawberries

1 kiwi (peeling optional)

½ mango

¼ cup lime juice

2 tablespoons agave nectar

PIÑA COLADA (high-protein)

1 cup coconut milk

½ cup 100% pineapple juice

1 banana

2 cups spinach

¼ cup pineapple

1 strawberry

¼ cup unsweetened coconut,
shredded or flakes

1 tablespoon protein powder

Dessert

Because even one day is too long to go without dessert, here are some no-cheat thick, creamy, sweet, low-calorie ways to smooth your way, even during the holiday season.

THANKSGIVING PUMPKIN PIE

1 cup coconut or nut milk

1 banana

2 cups fresh spinach

¾ cup pumpkin puree

3 pitted Medjool dates

¼ cup fresh or frozen cranberries

2 tablespoons ground pecans

1 teaspoon ground cinnamon

1 teaspoon ground pumpkin pie spice

DATE, HONEY, NUT NOT-A-MUFFIN (high-protein)

½ cup water

½ cup nut milk

2 bananas

1 cup Swiss chard

1 cup spinach

4 Medjool dates

¼ cup honey

¼ cup walnuts

¼ cup yogurt

1 teaspoon vanilla extract

pinch of ground cardamom

pinch of ground coriander

PEACHES 'N' CREAM (high-protein)

1 cup nut milk

1 banana

1 cup cabbage

¼ cup yogurt

1 cup spinach

2 peaches

2 teaspoons honey

BERRY BERRY PIE (high-protein)

1 cup almond milk

½ banana

2 cups spinach

½ cup blueberries

½ cup strawberries

1 tablespoon sesame seed

1 teaspoon poppy seeds

1 teaspoon vanilla extract

¼ cup almonds

½ cup yogurt

18 Smoothies for Your Daily Needs

PRE-WORKOUT (high-protein)

Pump up your workout with this high-energy smoothie.

1 cup water

½ apple

2 cups kale

¼ cup spirulina, wheat grass,
   or chlorella powder

¼ cup goji berries

2 tablespoons pumpkin seeds

½ cup soy milk

POST-WORKOUT (high-protein)

Jump-start your recovery with this hydrating, low-calorie, protein- and potassium heavy-green drink.

1½ cups water

1 banana

1 cup kale

1 cup spinach

1 cup strawberries

¼ cup cooked quinoa

½ cup nonfat Greek yogurt

1 tablespoon protein powder

KEEP IT SMOOTH: STOP THE CLOG

Give this green smoothie recipe a try for your constipation.

- 2 to 3 cups water
- 1 peach
- 2 cups any leafy green
- 1 avocado
- 2 carrots
- 2 pitted prunes
- ¼ cup presoaked steel-cut oatmeal
- 2 tablespoons ground flaxseed

KEEP IT SMOOTH: STOP THE TROTS (high-protein)

A green smoothie cleanse can work like Draino on your intestines. This smoothie will help prevent the runs.

- 1 cup water
- 1 banana
- 2 cups any leafy greens
- 1 apple
- 1 cup pitted cherries
- ¼ cup yogurt

"I HATE VEGETABLES" SMOOTHIE (high-protein)

You won't after whipping up this vat of green.

- 2 cups nut milk
- 1 banana
- 1 cup spinach
- 1 cup Napa cabbage
- ½ cup cauliflower
- 3 carrots
- 1 beet
- 1 red pepper
- 1 cup strawberries
- ½ cup blueberries
- 2 ounces dark chocolate
- 1 teaspoon vanilla extract
- 2 tablespoons spirulina

Super-Skinny Smoothie

Down these under-300-calorie drinks when you need to lose weight—or at least look like you have—by next weekend.

GINGER, OAT, AND BERRY BREAKFAST (200 calories)

1 cup water

1 banana

2 cups spinach

1 cup blackberries

½ cup strawberries

¼ cup presoaked steel-cut oatmeal

½ teaspoon grated fresh ginger

¼ cup nut milk

1 teaspoon honey

SOMETIMES YOU FEEL LIKE A NUT (250 calories; high-protein)

1 cup water

¼ cup nut milk

½ medium, ripe banana

2 cups spinach

1 cup raspberries

1 tablespoon peanut butter

SIMPLE SALAD LUNCH (162 calories; high-protein)

1 cup water

2 cups spinach

1½ cups chopped fresh honeydew

⅓ cup nonfat yogurt

COSMOPOLITAN COCKTAIL (220 calories)

1 cup 100% cranberry juice

¼ avocado

1 cup arugula

1 cup spinach

¼ cup dried cranberries

¼ cup fresh or frozen cranberries

2 tablespoons stevia or agave nectar

1 teaspoon lime juice

1 teaspoon lemon juice

FRUITY MULTIVITAMIN DINNER (192 calories; high-protein)

1 cup water

1 banana

1 cup raddichio

1 cup spinach

1 cup green grapes

½ Granny Smith apple

1 cup low-fat yogurt

MANGO, AVOCADO, AND LIME CREAM DREAM DESSERT (210 calories)

1 cup water

¼ cup avocado

2 cups spinach

1 cup mango

1 tablespoon lime juice

1 tablespoon fresh mint

1 teaspoon honey

THE MORNING AFTER SMOOTHIE

Mix this up when you need to kick-start your day after a tough night.

1 cup water

1 cup romaine lettuce

1 cup kale

1 banana

½ cucumber

2 asparagus ribs

1 cup watermelon

2 Medjool dates

1 tablespoon ground hemp seeds

½ tablespoon grated gingerroot

1 tablespoon goji berries

1 teaspoon spirulina

pinch of cayenne

MENSA SMOOTHIE (high-protein)

The ingredients in this green drink will juice your brain.

1 cup water

1 cup coconut water

1 cup kale

1 cup spinach

1 banana

½ cup strawberries

¼ cup almond butter

3 Brazil nuts

½ teaspoon vanilla extract

2 egg yolks or egg yolk powder

1 tablespoon cacao or cocoa powder

1 teaspoon ground cinnamon

MOOD BOOSTER (high-protein)

This smoothie has the right formula of minerals and vitamins to crank you right out of that bad mood.

½ cup water

½ cup 100% orange juice

2 bananas

2 cups spinach

1 cup watermelon

2 ounces tofu

1 tablespoon plain Greek yogurt

1 teaspoon lime juice

dash of grated ginger

1 teaspoon fresh mint

2 tablespoons agave nectar

YOU FORGOT TO SHOP SMOOTHIE

Use dandelion greens and any unsweetened canned fruit

LIME CUCUMBER PEAR SMOOTHIE

Slip into a white terry robe, stick your feet in a tub of warm, salted, scented water, and you will feel like you are at a spa as you sip this smoothie.

1 cup 100% apple juice

1 pear

1 cup loose-leaf lettuce

1 cup baby spinach

1 cucumber

1 bunch cilantro

1 bunch parsley

Green Smoothie Cleanse

BREATH FRESHENER

This will keep you Mentos-fresh all day.

1 cup water

1 banana

1 cup spinach

1 cup parsley

2 tablespoons chopped peppermint or spearmint leaves

Smoothie Upcycles

Tired of drinking? Here are five ways to make your smoothie and eat it!

- Green smoothie popsicles: Pour any smoothie into small Dixie cups with a stick and freeze.
- Pudding: Use a milk-based liquid such as nut milk or coconut milk and cut back the measurement to just ¼ cup; add 2 to 3 bananas to thicken the drink.
- Green smoothie fruit leather: Add 1 banana to thicken the smoothie; pour it into a dehydrator or onto a parchment-lined baking sheet and dry in a low oven (about 250°F) until dry but chewy.
- Green smoothie ice cream: Follow the same instructions as for pudding, but pour the smoothie into a 9 x 13-inch parchment-lined freezer-proof glass pan and freeze uncovered, stirring after 1 hour.
- Green smoothie soup: Pulse the ingredients until chunky instead of smooth and eat with a spoon.

Common Conversions

1 gallon = 4 quarts = 8 pints = 16 cups =128 fluid ounces = 3.8 liters
1 quart = 2 pints = 4 cups = 32 ounces = .95 liter
1 pint = 2 cups = 16 ounces = 480 ml
1 cup = 8 ounces = 240 ml
¼ cup = 4 tablespoons = 12 teaspoons = 2 ounces = 60 ml
1 tablespoon = 3 teaspoons = ½ fluid ounce = 15 ml

Temperature Conversions

FAHRENHEIT (°F)	CELSIUS (°C)
200°F	95°C
225°F	110°C
250°F	120°C
275°F	135°C
300°F	150°C
325°F	165°C
350°F	175°C
375°F	190°C
400°F	200°C
425°F	220°C
450°F	230°C
475°F	245°C

Volume Conversions

U.S.	U.S. EQUIVALENT	METRIC
1 teaspoon	½ fluid ounce	15 milliliters
1 tablespoon	2 fluid ounces	60 milliliters
1 cup	3 fluid ounces	90 milliliters
1 pint	4 fluid ounces	120 milliliters
1 quart	5 fluid ounces	150 milliliters
1 liter	6 fluid ounces	180 milliliters
1 ounce (dry)	8 fluid ounces	240 milliliters
1 pound	16 fluid ounces	480 milliliters

Weight Conversions

U.S.	METRIC
½ ounce	15 grams
1 ounce	30 grams
2 ounces	60 grams
¼ pound	115 grams
1/3 pound	150 grams
½ pound	225 grams
¾ pound	350 grams
1 pound	450 grams

Index

Food: chewing, 9; fresh vs. canned/ frozen, 40–42; shopping, 40–53; spoiled, 38–39; organic, 43, 46–48; swaps, 130. *See also* Fruits; Vegetables

Foods, fatty, 148; fermented, 147; fried, 148; low-fat, 155; processed, 127, 149–50; spoiled, 150

Free radicals, 19

Frozen foods, vs. fresh, 40–42

Frozen packaged meals, 156

Fruit/greens ratio, 14, 15, 100

Fruit leather, 241

Fruit/vegetable ratio, 26

Fruits: defined, 52–53; dried, 42; high fiber, 29; parts, 36–37, 63; and pesticides, 44–45, 47, 48–49; servings, 27; shopping, 40–53; speed-ripening, 49; spoiled, 38–39; storage, 49–50; as sweetener, 76; when to eat, 51–52

Full-Body Cleanse. *See* Two-Week Full-Body Cleanse

Gardening, 47

Gastric conditions, 24

Ginger root, 74, 80

Goals, 114–17

Goji berries, 71–72

Grains, whole, 79

Grapefruits, 48

Grapes, 45

Greek yogurt, recipe, 87

Green powder, 70–71

Green smoothie cleanses, in general, 94–104; goals, 114–17; and health problems, 20–24, 78–82; post-cleanse, 109; preparation, 122–40; programs, 111–21; strategies, 105–10. *See also specific cleanses*

Green smoothies: 94–104, 223–25; "add-ins," 62–92, 157–58, 211; benefits, 18–20; preparation, 49–51, 202–208

Greens (tops/leaves), 61

Greens/fruit ratio, 14, 15, 100

Gum, 7–8

Happy hour smoothies, 233–34

Hazelnuts, 73

Health problems, and green smoothies, 20–24, 78–82

Hemp seeds, 66

Herbs, fresh, 75

High blood pressure, 21–23

High-fructose corn syrup, 152–53

Honey, 76

Hydration. *See* Water

Ice cream, 241

Immune system, 95

Insoluble fiber, 24, 28, 57

Iodine, 37

Iron, 37–38, 57